# The Complete Book Of
# Questions
## Dog Owners Ask Their Vet
# &Answers

### By Dr. Steven Radbill
#### with Morris Kennedy

### Illustration by Suzanne Clee

RUNNING PRESS
PHILADELPHIA, PENNSYLVANIA

Canadian representatives: John Wiley & Sons Canada, Ltd.
22 Worcester Road, Rexdale, Ontario M9W 1L1

International representatives: Kaiman & Polon, Inc.
2175 Lemoine Avenue, Fort Lee, New Jersey 07024

9    8    7    6    5    4    3    2    1

Digit on the right indicates the number of this printing.

LIBRARY OF CONGRESS CATALOGING IN PUBLICATION DATA
Radbill, Steven, 1948-
The complete book of questions dog owners ask their vet.
Bibliography: p. 136
Includes index.
SUMMARY: A veterinarian discusses the selection,
training, care, breeds, and illnesses of dogs and
common myths about them. Includes a section of
emergency first aid procedures.
1. Dogs—Miscellanea.    2. Dogs—Diseases—Miscellanea.
[1. Dogs—Miscellanea.    2. Questions and answers]
I. Kennedy, Morris, joint author.    II. Title.
SF427.R23          636.7          79-20981
ISBN 0-89471-084-2 library binding
ISBN 0-89471-081-8 paperback

*Editor: Alida Becker*
*Cover art direction: James Wizard Wilson*
*Front cover photography: Carl Waltzer*
*Back cover photography: Burt Murtaugh*
*Interior design: Peter John Dorman*

*Typography: Caledonia, with Tiffany, by rci, Philadelphia, Pennsylvania*
*Printed and bound by Port City Press, Baltimore, Maryland*

This book may be ordered directly from the publisher.
Please include 50 cents postage.

**Try your bookstore first.**

Running Press
38 South Nineteenth Street
Philadelphia, Pennsylvania 19103

# INTRODUCTION

*Money will buy a pretty good dog, but it won't buy the wag of his tail.*
—Josh Billings

For thousands of years, human beings and dogs have enjoyed one of nature's most successful symbiotic relationships. Our part of the bargain is to provide food, shelter, and good care—and the training that can make a dog not only a source of companionship, but a reliable work and sport animal as well. On the surface, this might seem to be a simple matter, but it can become awfully complicated. We hope this book will take some of the guesswork out of raising and caring for your dog, and we've included all the questions you're liable to ask—from the time you think about picking out a dog, through the challenging times when you're training your dog, all the way to the special problems you're likely to face when your dog grows older. You'll also learn about day-to-day care; and when your dog has health problems, you can turn to the troubleshooting segment of the book, where the questions are keyed to specific symptoms and their implications. Emergency situations are also covered in a comprehensive first aid section.

All the questions are numbered consecutively and grouped into six basic categories that are further subdivided so you can turn quickly to the entry you need. When there's related information elsewhere in the book, the number of the question in which it can be found is listed as a cross reference in parentheses. A complete index at the back of the book is also arranged by question number, and the annotated bibliography that appears at the beginning of the Appendix can suggest other sources if you're interested in further reading.

We'd like to note, in passing, that we've decided to refer throughout the book to our canine friends by using personal pronouns. It's not terribly clinical, but we think it's a more natural expression of our relationships with our pets. In most cases, the use of the personal pronoun in any particular question and answer is purely arbitrary.

This book is designed to help you give your dog the right kind of care—and an important part of that care is the ability to recognize what problems can be treated at home and what problems need professional attention. Picking a verterinarian is the most important decision you'll make for your dog. When you go to a clinic for the first time, consider the quality of the examination your animal is given. Is it thorough and careful, or rushed? Does the vet explain what he or she is doing and what's wrong with the dog? Remember, elaborate equipment isn't as important as the little things. Is the clinic clean? Is the staff friendly? Does the vet tell you what you should expect from the drugs being prescribed and what each pill is for? If there's anything you don't understand, ask questions. After all, it takes cooperation and trust between you and your veterinarian to insure your dog of the best possible care. We hope the information provided in this book will help you toward that end.

*Dr. Steven S. Radbill*
and *Morris Kennedy*
*Philadelphia, 1980*

# TABLE OF CONTENTS

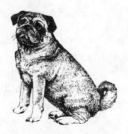

## PART I
## CARING FOR YOUR DOG

Choosing a Dog
*page 11*

Caring for a Puppy
*page 16*

Training a Puppy
*page 21*

Feeding
*page 24*

Grooming
*page 30*

Caring for Nails, Ears, and Teeth
*page 33*

Dog Paraphernalia
*page 37*

Exercise
*page 40*

Travel and Boarding
*page 42*

The Older Dog
*page 44*

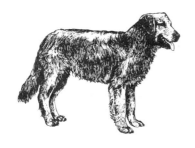 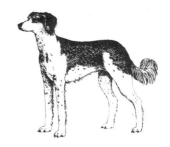

## PART II
# UNDERSTANDING YOUR DOG

Dogs and Children
*page 49*

The Problem Dog
*page 51*

Dog Facts: Popular Beliefs, Common Behavior
*page 58*

The Dog's Body and How It Works
*page 60*

## PART III
# GENERAL MEDICAL CARE

Preventive Medicine: Monitoring Your Dog's Health
*page 65*

Home Medical Care
*page 67*

Spaying and Castration
*page 72*

PART IV

# BREEDING

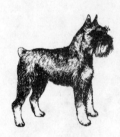

Mating and Reproduction
*page 76*

Pregnancy and Birth
*page 79*

Caring for the Mother and Her Pups
*page 85*

Weaning
*page 90*

PART V

# ACCIDENTS AND AILMENTS

First Aid
*page 93*

Common Ailments: Vomiting, Diarrhea, Constipation
*page 104*

Eye, Ear, and Mouth Problems
*page 107*

Respiratory Ailments
*page 109*

Skin Conditions, Abscesses, Sores
*page 111*

Muscle and Bone Problems
*page 113*

External Parasites
*page 115*

Internal Parasites
*page 119*

Miscellaneous Ailments
*page 123*

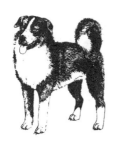 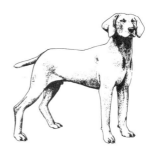

PART VI
# SERIOUS ILLNESSES

Hip Dysplasia
*page 125*

Distemper
*page 126*

Rabies
*page 127*

Heart Disease
*page 128*

Cancer
*page 129*

Other Serious Illnesses
*page 130*

Euthanasia
*page 133*

# APPENDIX

Annotated Bibliography • A First Aid Kit For Your Dog
Your Dog's Medical Record
*pages 136-140*

# INDEX
*page 141*

# PART I

# CARING FOR YOUR DOG

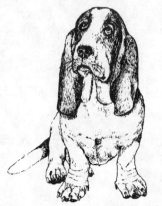

*Basset Hound*

### Choosing a Dog
1-27

### Caring for a Puppy
28-55

### Training a Puppy
56-68

### Feeding
69-99

### Grooming
100-118

### Caring for Nails, Ears, and Teeth
119-141

### Dog Paraphernalia
142-157

### Exercise
158-168

### Travel and Boarding
169-179

### The Older Dog
180-192

# Choosing a Dog

*1. Do you recommend any particular breed for people who live in the city—or the country?*  Small breeds, such as toys, are generally well suited for someone who lives in a city apartment or travels a great deal. However, they can be quite noisy, and they don't adapt well to small children. Some of the most popular small breeds are the toy poodle, the Chihuahua, the pug, and the Yorkshire terrier. If you prefer a slightly larger dog that adapts well to city life, a miniature poodle, cocker spaniel, Lhasa apso, or cairn terrier may be what you need. A *large* dog that's temperamentally suited to life in the city is the German shepherd, which can get along with no trouble at all, provided you have enough room in your apartment and a little bit of a yard. Probably the *worst* dog for close city living is the Irish setter. This dog needs plenty of running space and is miserable if it's cooped up. If you have plenty of space and are the outdoor type, setters and other sporting breeds such as springer spaniels and pointers make excellent companions. Obviously, when you don't live in the city you have many more options when it comes to picking out a dog—the breeds I've mentioned are just a few of the dozens you might choose from. If you're thinking about getting a purebred dog, it makes sense to take the time to familiarize yourself with the different breeds before you select one (193). The best way to do that is to visit dog shows, talk to as many breeders as you can, and read up on the subject.

*2. What kind of expense am I getting into when I buy a dog?*  Beyond the initial cost of the dog, which could range from a nominal fee at a shelter to hundreds of dollars at a breeder's, you'll have to buy dog food and some equipment, such as a collar and a leash. You'll also have to pay license fees of about five or ten dollars, as well as the charges for regular, annual veterinary examinations and shots. Other possible expenses include professional grooming (114) and any emergency medical treatment. The first year's medical costs, including neutering and shots, should be between $100 and $150. After that, yearly expenses for health maintenance and shots should be no more than about $50. All of these expenses will vary from dog to dog, but this run-down will give you some idea of what to expect.

*3. What advantages are there in getting a purebred dog?*  By buying a purebred dog you can, in effect, tailor your dog to your own tastes and environment. If you see a dog you like, very often you can go to the same breeder and get an animal from the same bloodline, so that even minor characteristics can be selected in advance. There's also the major advantage of knowing what the puppies will be like if you decide to breed your dog. It's also much easier to find homes for purebred pups, which can be quite valuable. Of course, there *are* some problems with purebreds that are the result of inbreeding over the years. A thorough check of the dog's lineage and a physical examination can safeguard against many of these genetic problems.

*4. Is a purebred dog more temperamental than a mutt?*  This is a kind of folk, animal-psychology notion, and it just isn't true. Some dogs are crazy, some moody or grumpy, and some particular about what they eat, but it doesn't matter whether they're purebred or mongrels. It *is* true that certain breeds have their own general personality traits, but the spectrum of breeds is so wide that you can't flatly declare that purebreds as such have any particular temperament.

**5. *What's the best place to buy a dog?*** If you're looking for a top-of-the-line show dog and you want to make sure that genetic problems have been eliminated as much as possible, your best bet is a private breeder. If you don't know any breeders, you can start by looking in a dog magazine (there are even some that specialize in certain breeds), checking with local veterinarians for recommendations, and talking with people who own dogs you especially like. You can also ask about a breeder at the local kennel club or dog fanciers' association. You'll find that dog shows and obedience trials are also good places to make contacts and pick up information. When you pick a breeder, it's to your advantage to buy from someone nearby—if all the other factors are equal. A local breeder can be more accessible if you have problems with the dog, and the breeder's references will be easier to check. If show qualities don't matter to you, and you just want an affectionate, good-tempered animal, I recommend that you try to find a dog in a private home. In most cases, the puppy will have had lots of petting and human contact, which is crucial in developing a good family pet. Another possibility that's attractive to real bargain hunters is the local animal shelter (9).

**6. *Do you recommend getting a dog from a pet shop?*** You may be taking quite a risk. The animals might have been shipped in from a puppy "factory," a mass-production animal farm where dogs are bred simply for resale, with no particular regard for genetic problems, temperament, or the fine points of breeding. Another disadvantage of pet-shop dogs is that they often have very little human contact, which can make them withdrawn and hard to train. Their environment can also be physically harmful because the animals are more apt to be exposed to communicable diseases. If you shop at a pet store, make certain the dealer gives a lifetime guarantee against inherited disorders such as hip dysplasia and collie eye syndrome. These traits can show up *years* after the dog leaves the store and can only be prevented through selective breeding. A reputable dealer should have such a policy.

**7. *If a puppy turns out to be unhealthy, or otherwise unsatisfactory, can it be returned?*** Usually you'll be allowed to exchange an unwanted animal within a time limit of at least 72 hours, which gives you a chance to have the dog checked over by a veterinarian. Pet stores often allow as long as a week for a buyer to decide whether or not to keep a dog. The prospect of getting a full refund is a lot less likely than a simple exchange, so be sure you know what the breeder or pet store's policy is *before* you agree to buy a dog.

**8. *Is there a difference between crossbreeds and mixed breeds?*** The American Kennel Club is the final authority on what constitutes a breed, and if a dog isn't purebred and registered as such, the animal is a mixed breed, even if the two strains the dog comes from are purebred. In buying a "crossbreed" dog, you know a little more about what kind of dog the puppy will become than you would if you bought a mongrel, but these dogs don't constitute a *new* breed.

**9. *What's a good place to get a mixed breed dog?*** The obvious choice—your local animal shelter. They'll usually have a wide selection of pups to choose from, and they can always use help in finding a home for their dogs. Make sure you ask lots of questions: What size will the puppy be when he's fully grown? Why was the puppy turned over to a shelter? Has he had any vaccinations? How has he been eating?

What does his temperament seem to be like? Take the pup out of the cage and see how he approaches you. If you have children, bring them along and make sure they get to handle the pup too. You could also try answering any interesting ads in the newspaper. This can be a good way to pick out a pup because you'll be able to see the mother and the father, and some of the other members of the litter. You'll be able to get a better idea of the size a pup will grow to, and what sort of temperament he'll have. A pup from a private home will be less likely to have personality problems because of his early contact with people and the good care he's been given.

*10. What are the drawbacks and benefits to think about when I'm choosing between a male and a female dog?* Either sex can be very affectionate and good with children, providing the dog is brought up properly. And neither sex has an advantage over the other where overall health is concerned. Males *do* tend to be more aggressive, especially with other males, and sometimes this comes out in the way they act toward people. Females are less likely to roam around; they're easier to train and more obedient; females also seem less inclined to be hyperactive. On the other hand, a female dog will go into heat twice a year if you don't have her spayed.

*11. What should I keep in mind when I'm choosing between a longhaired dog and a shorthaired one?* There are four main things to consider: the climate of the area you live in, how great its flea and tick problem is, the time you can spend grooming the dog, and the problems that can be caused by shedding. Naturally, a dog that's adapted to cold, northern climates will suffer quite a bit in tropical climates. Shorthaired dogs have an advantage where fleas and ticks are concerned because they offer these parasites less protection from pesticides and other control methods. You should also make your decision based on the amount of time you're willing to spend grooming your dog (100). Finally, you should consider the amount of aggravation that shedding might cause your family (23).

*12. What signs of good or bad health should I look for when I'm picking out a puppy?* First, check her eyes and nose to make sure they're free of discharges or redness; these are the early signs of an upper respiratory infection or even distemper. The ears should be clean and have no strong, unpleasant odor about them; waxy discharge in the ear and a bad smell are the signs of an ear infection. Pick up a pinch of skin on the puppy's back, and then release it; the flesh should return quickly to its original shape. If it doesn't, the dog could be dehydrated, a symptom of any number of illnesses and a sign that the puppy hasn't been eating or taking water properly for three or four days. Dandruff and dryness of the coat are further indications of long-standing illness; if the animal is healthy her coat should be full and shiny. A pot-bellied stomach will tell you that the dog probably has worms; and pale, cold gums are a sign of some problem involving a loss of blood. Of course, in addition to these specific physical indicators, the puppy should be active and alert.

*13. What are some good clues to a puppy's personality and temperament?* When you approach the pup he shouldn't back away or snarl. He should come to you freely, provided you don't do something to frighten him. Pick up the puppy (14) and see how he responds. A certain amount of squirming is to be expected at first, but if the dog becomes very excited and tries hard to wiggle free, he may be hyperactive or overly sensitive to being touched. A puppy that's unaccustomed to human contact will often cry when he's picked up; such a dog may have trouble developing a bond with people or be hand-shy, distant, and hard to train. If the puppy cries and whines when he experiences a mild amount of rough handling, you'd do well to choose another dog. Likewise, be cautious of a puppy that plays *too* hard, one that becomes very aggressive and excited. Instead, look for a puppy that's alert and curious; he should be playful, but not in a nervous, uncontrollable way. It's also helpful to watch how a pup treats his littermates; by the time they're ready for adoption, they'll already have established a social order. The dominant pup will usually boss the others around, and the most submissive one will cower. Try to select a pup whose behavior falls *between* those two extremes, and you'll have a dog that's easier to train and discipline, one with a more gentle, pleasing personality.

**14. How should I hold a puppy when I pick her up?** Support the puppy's hind end with one hand and put the other hand under her chest. If you always try to support a pup's hind end, the animal will feel more secure and be less inclined to squirm around and try to break free. Always be gentle with a puppy, and never try to pick her up by the scruff of the neck only.

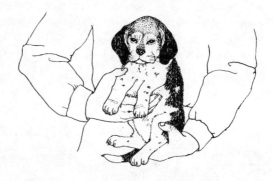

**15. What's the best age to bring home a puppy?** Between eight and twelve weeks, a pup begins to be more interested in the outside world and is more likely to react well with and form strong attachments to people. Obviously, that's the best time to introduce the animal into your household. No dog under six weeks old should be separated from her mother and littermates. The pup may not be properly weaned, and she can develop health problems from a lack of proper nutrition. In addition to this, the pup will tend to become too attached to people, not only because she lacks maturity but also because she missed the socialization to other dogs that she would have gotten by being with her brothers and sisters. All this can make a puppy overly dependent on her master, a situation that can be very distressing to the dog and annoying to the people around her. At the other extreme is the dog that's taken by an owner too late, after she's about sixteen weeks old. You won't have any difficulty adopting an older puppy, as long as she's been kept by a family and given plenty of attention. But if the dog has been alone, perhaps caged, since she was weaned, as is the case with many kennel and pet shop dogs, she will already be developing a pattern of withdrawal from human beings and could have some difficult behavioral problems. The training that involves confinement in a cage (50) is wasted on a dog like this because the animal has spent most or all of its life in a cage anyway.

**16. Is there any particular season that's best for getting a new puppy?** That's mostly up to you. It should be a season when you, or someone in the family, will be home almost all of the time, so that the dog has plenty of companionship and opportunities for training and supervision. The only other consideration is the weather. Warm weather is preferable because the young puppy will be able to have plenty of access to the outdoors for housebreaking, exercise, and exploration. There's also less chance that the pup will develop health problems from exposure to cold, or become bored from being indoors for long stretches.

**17. *Can you tell how big a puppy will grow to be by looking at the size of his paws?*** Most of the time, this is a fairly good indicator—big paws are usually a sign that you'll wind up with a big *dog*. For another clue, look just above the paw for the bump where the dog's wrist will be. This is the growth plate of the pup's leg bones; the bone will grow upward from this point. If the pup will be very large when he's fully grown, this plate will be quite prominent.

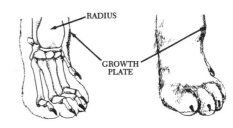

**18. *Does the color of a puppy's coat sometimes change after he gets older?*** The fuzziness of a puppy's coat goes away when he's about six months old, and this can change the color. Within some breeds, there's also a natural shift in the color of the coat as the dog matures, but it's nothing extreme, and usually predictable.

**19. *Should I get a puppy if nobody is home during the day?*** This isn't a good idea. Without plenty of personal contact early in life, a dog often grows up to become a very neurotic, troublesome pet. When a puppy is eight weeks old, he's learning some key lessons in socialization with people. If the pup doesn't have a lot of interaction with humans during this time, he can become a real problem later on—constantly seeking attention, barking, destroying things, and so on. If you want a dog, why not consider an adult? There are almost always plenty of well-adjusted, grown dogs at the animal shelter that would adapt nicely to your situation.

**20. *What should I look for when I'm picking out an older dog?*** It's important to know that an older dog has been raised with a lot of human contact and affection. A dog that was isolated from people during the first few months of his life will be more likely to have some behavioral problems that will be hard to change, but if the dog is well trained and affectionate, there shouldn't be any difficulty.

**21. *Is it a good idea to get a dog if you have very small children?*** With the right selection, either a purebred or a mixed breed dog can become an important part of your child's early education. Make sure that the child is at least two before you bring a new dog into the household; this way he or she will already have some understanding of what a dog is and how to approach him (197). Make sure to choose a dog with a calm temperament, one that's obedient and doesn't snap easily (193).

**22. *Should I take my child to pick out a new dog?*** Yes, if the youngster is old enough—say, over five years old. After all, you'll want to see how the child and the dog interact to make sure you get a dog that isn't afraid of children and will take to handling by a child. It's also just a nice thing to do. The dog is going to be your son's or daughter's pet, and the child should be there for the selection. Watch the child and the dog carefully—if the dog shies away from the child and cowers, choose another one. The same thing applies to a dog that snarls and barks with hostility, and also to the hyperactive dog, which may tend to nip and knock down a child and play too aggressively. You should make the final decision, but a child who's old enough to make a reasonable choice shouldn't be left out of it.

**23. What's the best breed for a person who has allergies?**  Wirehaired dogs such as poodles, terriers, and schnauzers are the best choice. They shed very little and have hardly any dander (the flakes from skin ailments) that can serve as an irritant.

**24. We want a second dog. Should we get one that's the same sex as the one we have now?**  Two females will usually get along with no trouble. Two males, on the other hand, tend to compete too much and are apt to be hard to handle. Of course, if you have a pair, one will have to be neutered—unless you want puppies by them or you're able to keep them isolated when the female is in heat.

**25. Is there anything we can do to help smooth the way when we get a second dog?**  When a second dog comes into a household, especially if the dog is a young puppy, the new dog will almost always be submissive to the dog in residence (29). This dominance ranking may change in the future, but you shouldn't try to influence the social order between the dogs. People tend to feel that dogs should be very democratic and coexist as equals, but this isn't the way dogs operate. Any two dogs that are thrown together for more than a few minutes will establish a dominant-submissive arrangement with each other, and the two will be content with this as long as the owner doesn't foster competition unnecessarily. When you bring in a new dog, pay more attention to your *old* dog so that you don't create resentment between the two animals.

**26. Will our cat get along with a new dog?**  Kittens and puppies are usually excellent companions, but an adult cat that has spent a lot of time indoors with little or no contact with other animals may not like a new dog in the house. A good way of telling how your cat will respond to a new dog is to have someone bring a dog to your house for a visit to give you a chance to see how the cat acts. Usually a household with more than one cat will have no difficulty taking in a new dog.

**27. I need a good watchdog to protect my house. What breed do you recommend?**  What most people are after in a watchdog is an animal that knows when to bark. A dog's ability to *bite* isn't much protection against a well-prepared burglar, who will either pacify or kill the dog if he has to. On the other hand, many burglars will pass up a house with a loud dog, since there are plenty of quieter houses to choose from. Just be sure to get yourself a *pet*, the kind of dog you'll be happy with during all those days and hours when he isn't chasing away criminals. If you *really* want a full-fledged guard dog, get one that's been professionally trained. The breeds used for this job are well known—Doberman pinschers and German shepherds, for the most part. Training is of key importance when you're getting a guard dog. You'll want a dog that's obedient and intelligent, not just one that attacks strangers.

## Caring for a Puppy

**28. How should I prepare for the pup's homecoming?**  Be sure that you can spend plenty of time with the pup while he's getting used to his new home. The ideal time would be a long weekend or during your vacation. Make sure to prepare a permanent place for the pup to sleep and rest; most people prefer to use a small area in the kitchen or a large box. Keep in mind the fact that changes can be traumatic for a dog, and one of the ways a puppy responds to stress is to stop eating. Don't be surprised if the pup doesn't eat for the first day or so, but if this continues for more than 48 hours you should contact your veterinarian. While we're on the subject, it's also important to find out what the pup's been fed and keep him on the same diet for at least the first couple of days. Later on, you can introduce new foods, but if you change the diet too abruptly the puppy is apt to get diarrhea.

*29.  What's the best way to introduce a new puppy to our other dog?*   To begin with, don't let the puppy have free reign of the house. The old dog has an established territory there, and it isn't fair to let the pup move into it suddenly. This could also cause some dangerous fights. When first introducing the two, you should be with the adult dog, and call the puppy over. This way the adult dog doesn't feel slighted and become jealous (25, 191). If the two dogs are pleased with each other's company and play, let them get acquainted, but for the first two weeks make sure they're together *only* in your presence. Watch how the dogs interact, and if the puppy becomes rambunctious and annoys the older dog, try to discipline it; put the pup out of the way while you remain with the older dog. Later on, you can bring them back together. Continue these supervised and controlled encounters until the dogs get used to each other and establish a social order. Sometimes an adult male and a male puppy will get along very nicely until the pup gets to be about six months old and begins to try to exert dominance. When this happens, fights can result, and you should consider having the pup castrated. It's always better to castrate the submissive dog of a pair. Castrating the dominant dog will possibly only put the dogs on an *even* social level, creating a constant state of tension.

*30.  When should I take the pup to the vet?*   Wait about two days and use that time to keep an eye on the puppy's eating and drinking habits, his bowel movements, and his activity in general (7). This way you'll have some history to present to the vet so that he or she can come up with an accurate diagnosis as to the pup's general health. Remember to take along a stool sample on this first trip so that the vet can check for worms.

*31.  How can I tell if our new puppy has worms?*   The worm that's most common in pups is roundworm. Pups can get roundworms even before they're born, while in their mother's womb, or later from her milk. The signs of a roundworm infestation are coughing, diarrhea, vomiting, a potbellied appearance, and a dull-looking coat. You may also notice that the pup will be moaning from her belly pains and will seem to be very uncomfortable. Sometimes you can see the worms in the dog's feces or in her vomit; the worms will be two to three inches long and white, and they'll tend to curl up. The best way to tell if your pup has worms is to take a stool sample to your vet.

*32.  How old does my puppy have to be before I can treat him for roundworms?*   This can usually be taken care of when the pups are getting their first vaccinations, at the age of six weeks. They need three doses of wormer, administered at ten-day intervals (579). Unless the infestation is particularly bad, it's an easy thing to cure.

**33. What should I feed my puppy?**  It's best to feed a fully weaned puppy a combination of half dry food and half canned puppy food. Puppies need a dry food that has a 20 to 27% protein content; the label should read "nutritionally complete for puppies" (70). Canned food has less protein but it's high in calories and fat, both of which the pup needs. Dry food will round out the diet by providing protein, vitamins A and D, calcium, and phosphorus (81). If you only give the pup dry food, be sure to add a teaspoon of cooking oil every day. Your pup needs this for his coat.

**34. How often should I feed my puppy?**  From age six to twelve weeks, feed the pup three times a day. After twelve weeks, cut back to twice a day until the dog is six months old. Then feed her once a day.

**35. About how much food should I give our new puppy so that she grows, but doesn't get fat?**  A small dog needs a meal that consists of about three tablespoons of canned food and a quarter of a cup of dry food, medium-sized pups need five tablespoons of canned food to a third of a cup of dry, and large breeds can eat one third to half a can of food and a half a cup of dry food. The morning meal should be lighter; the evening meal should be the largest. Watch how the puppy eats, and if she still seems hungry after a meal, increase the portion during the next meal by about 20% and see if that fills her up. As the dog grows, the amount of food should increase accordingly.

**36. Should I give my puppy milk?**  It's usually not a good idea because ordinary milk can cause diarrhea. One way to avoid this is to try mixing in some low-fat or powdered milk with the dog's food.

**37. Is it all right to feed my puppy eggs?**  Yes. Eggs are especially good for the pup's coat. Give a small puppy an average of three eggs a week; six is fine for larger puppies. The egg can be cooked or raw, whichever the pup prefers.

**39. Are there any toys that you recommend specifically for puppies?**  The same standards apply for dogs of all ages—hard-rubber toys are good, and so are rawhide chews, as long as they're large enough so they can't be broken up and eaten. Don't get the pup too many toys—no more than about three (62)—and stay away from latex toys with squeakers inside them that can be torn up and swallowed (155).

**40. What kind of collar do you recommend for a puppy?**  There's a combination collar and training leash that's good for breaking a pup in to walking on a leash. It's a strip of nylon with a loop at each end. When you use it, just keep constant but light pressure on the pup's neck. Lead him around gently and keep him at your side, but don't use force until the dog is five or six months old (226). You can get him a permanent leather collar when he's four months old. Remember, though, that the dog will still be growing at that age. A collar should be loose enough to move freely on your dog's neck and allow room for your fingers beneath it, but it should be tight enough not to slip off over the dog's head.

**41. Do you recommend having a puppy tattooed for identification?**  Yes, especially if the dog is very valuable. In the case of a theft or a dispute over a lost dog, the tattoo may be the only thing you can use to prove that the dog belongs to you. Animal shelters usually do this for a small fee; the dog is marked on the belly or the ear.

**42. When should a puppy get a license?**   A dog is licensed after the animal is six months old, at the time of the first rabies shot. In some areas, you'll be given a discount on the license fee if the dog is castrated or spayed.

**43. We just bought a puppy from a kennel, and she seems weak and sickly now. Could she have picked up something around the other dogs?**   A number of diseases can be passed from dog to dog in a poorly managed kennel. If the pup has a raspy, wrenching cough she may have tracheobronchitis, an easily treatable respiratory illness (523). If she becomes worse and begins vomiting, has severe diarrhea, and if her nose and eyes drain with mucus, this could be distemper, a much more serious ailment (608). The odds are, though, that your pup has coccidiosis, one of the most common diseases puppies bring home with them from a crowded kennel. It's caused by a one-celled organism called a coccidium, and its symptoms are heavy diarrhea, a dull coat, slight anemia, and a poor appetite. A very mild infection might have little or no outward signs at all, but the disease can weaken a dog and leave her vulnerable to other illnesses. Antibiotics are used to eliminate the infection. Coccidiosis does occasionally affect older dogs, but they tend to develop a resistance to it over the years.

**44. What causes a puppy's stomach to break out in pimple-like bumps?**   Any one of a number of minor skin infections can create a patch that looks like acne on the puppy's belly. It should clear up with a swabbing of mild antiseptic solution or alcohol twice a day. Try that for three days, and if there's no change you'll probably need to go to your vet for antibiotics.

**45. How much should a healthy puppy sleep?**   This varies a good deal. Young puppies sleep quite a bit, and any dog will sleep after a meal—so pups that are eating three times a day will naturally take a lot of naps. When the pup is eight weeks old, he should begin to be very lively, but he'll still take frequent short naps. Don't worry about the pup's sleeping habits unless he's very hard to rouse, seems lethargic, and can't play longer than about fifteen minutes without getting tired. This could be a sign of illness and should be investigated by your veterinarian.

**46. When does a puppy go through teething?**   There's no such thing as "teething" in puppies; they don't suffer any teething pain the way human babies do. They have all their baby teeth by the time they're eight weeks old, and they lose them gradually; all the permanent teeth will be in place by the time the dog is six months old. The teeth fall out periodically, and sometimes you'll notice one on the floor. This is nothing to be alarmed about. Just make sure the puppy has a toy to chew on, and that she doesn't get into the habit of chewing on other things (62).

**47. How much handling should a young puppy have? Is it possible to handle a puppy too much?**   Actually, it's been found that handling is very *good* for the puppy. But make sure you do it *gently*. Don't force the puppy; handle him carefully and let him down when he's tired of playing (425).

*48. How do I get my pup used to general grooming, such as cutting his nails and brushing him?* This has to be started *early*, even as early as the first week you have the pup. You should take a lot of care not to frighten the animal (425). Get a good nail clipper from your local pet store and stroke the pup as you work, keeping him calm, but holding him firmly. Cut his nails beyond the red part where the vein is, just clipping off the small points (119). Remember that you don't have to do all ten front toes at once. It's fine to do one or two a day until you get them all clipped. The same goes for using the brush (101). Just give the pup a few gentle strokes at a time.

*49. Should the puppy be allowed to explore the house or should she be confined?* It's generally a good idea to let the pup explore the house—but only under your supervision. Be sure to do this gradually, and always when you're there to keep an eye on things. The puppy should *never* be given free reign of the house at night. When you go to bed she should be confined to her sleeping area.

*50. How large a space should I set aside for the puppy?* Generally, the best way to confine the pup is to use a collapsible cagelike enclosure; the standard ones usually measure about $2 \times 4$ feet and stand about 3 feet high. These are fine for a pup that's not going to grow too big (about 30 lbs.); for a pup that's going to grow larger, obviously you'll need a larger cage. Most people think that caging a dog is awful, but it's actually extremely beneficial. Once the pup gets used to the area, he'll grow to enjoy it and use it as his own "room" in the house.

*51. How should I introduce the puppy to his cage?* You shouldn't just throw him in and keep him locked up for eight hours at a time, or even for the whole night. When you first bring him home, put him in the cage for ten or fifteen minutes at a time. Usually any young dog, when isolated like this, will cry and bark and yowl, but if you introduce him to the cage at ten or fifteen minute intervals, leave him, and then come and get him, he'll generally settle down. The most important point to remember is that if you leave the puppy unattended, not in his own crate or den, he's going to feel the isolation even more, and may react with destructive behavior. By confining the puppy, you're going to help *prevent* this kind of activity. By the time he's six to eight months old, he'll be much less likely to form bad habits, and you'll be able to give him a freer reign in the house.

*52. How can I make the puppy comfortable in her cage?* It helps to put a blanket over the cage to make it more like a den. It also helps to feed the puppy while she's in the cage. On the first day, put the food right outside the cage, then move it inside on the second or third day, after the pup has become accustomed to eating at the cage. Another good idea is to put some article of your clothing in the enclosure. Dogs make most of their associations by scent instead of sight, so if you put something that smells like you in the cage, the pup will be more at ease.

*53. Will a pup feel more comfortable in a new home if you put a clock in her cage?* This myth is based on the idea that the pup will think the ticking clock is mother's heartbeat. Dogs are too smart to be fooled by a cheap trick like that.

*54. What should I do if my puppy carries on and barks and cries all night in the cage?* If the pup keeps on barking and just won't settle down in the cage, you can try putting the crate in your bedroom at night for the first week or two. This will give your puppy enough social contact so that he'll be comfortable and calm down. After that, you can gradually move him out of the room. Another important thing to remember is that the time when the puppy is crying to get out is *not* the time to let him out. Have him calm down first and *then* let him out. If you release him when he cries, he's going to learn that crying will get him out—and he'll continue to do it. Instead, scold him slightly, not too harshly, and then let him out when he quiets down. Don't make a big fuss when you release him, just let him quietly out of the cage—the idea is *not* to give him the impression he's being rewarded.

**55. *When can a puppy start spending time outside alone?*** No dog should be outside alone until he's three months old (158). Then, provided the weather is mild, let the dog stay outside for a couple of hours, and gradually increase the time he's alone over the weeks that follow. By the time the dog is about six months old, it should be safe to leave the animal outside for a full day. Of course, no dog should ever be allowed to roam; if the dog is outside he should be within a fence or on a chain or a leash.

## Training a Puppy

**56. *Is it okay to hit the pup to discipline him?*** Generally speaking, no. This usually makes him very hand-shy, and he'll also learn to cower when you approach. The best way to discipline the pup if you catch him in the act—eliminating in the house, chewing on something, tipping over the trash, barking excessively, etc.—is simply to grab him by the scruff of the neck, shake him gently, and praise him when he stops the bad behavior. Another technique is to make a loud noise. Get a can, fill it with beebees or something that will make a sharp noise, and just shake it. This is a very unpleasant noise for the animal, and he'll generally stop what he's been doing.

**57. *How do I keep my pup from barking so much?*** The easiest way to cut down on barking is to make sure not to *teach* your dog to bark. In other words, don't teach her to bark for food or to bark when she wants to go outside. Use behavior modification techniques whenever this happens. Tell your dog to stop in a loud, firm voice. Many dogs tend to bark when people come to your front door, and this isn't generally a good idea unless your dog has been trained as a guard dog. Otherwise, you're not going to be able to control the dog's barking at all and it can become quite a nuisance. It's better to train her to bark when someone approaches, but to stop on command. To teach her this, grab her by the scruff of the neck, shake her gently, and command her to stop barking. Also, make sure your dog doesn't get in the habit of barking at noises that she hears *outside*. This can be annoying to your neighbors— especially when you're not home. If you have this problem and you're going to be leaving the dog alone in the house, it's a good idea to leave a radio on. This will mask some of the sounds she might hear from the outside (223).

**58. *Our puppy seems very quiet, and we want her to be a good watchdog. Should we encourage her to bark?*** Teaching a dog to bark can bring out the animal's aggressive tendencies, and these can develop into behavioral problems when the animal gets older. The dog will learn to bark on her own, instinctively, and will usually do so in defending her territory (and your house). At the most, you could very judiciously praise a particularly quiet young dog when there's a situation in which you want the dog to bark—for example, if there's a prowler around. But you should also make it clear when you want the dog to *stop*. A bit of advice from a professional trainer can also be helpful.

**59. How should I housebreak my new puppy?**   One of the first rules of housebreaking is to feed your puppy at *specific* times. Don't leave food out all the time. Your pup will usually have a bowel movement about fifteen minutes to half an hour after meals, and that's when you should take her out for her walk. Always try to use the same door when you take the dog outside—that way, the dog will learn to go there when she needs to be walked. Try to take her to the same spot every time because this spot will be scented, and the scent will encourage her to eliminate in the area. After she has eliminated, praise the pup highly, speaking in a soft voice. Praising her whenever she eliminates in the proper place will reinforce the behavior pattern. As a general rule, you should take the pup out shortly after she eats, drinks, takes a nap, plays, or any time she looks restless. For the first couple of weeks, you might be taking her out as often as ten or twelve times a day, but after that you'll learn her routine and you shouldn't have to take her out more than five or six times a day.

**60. Should I train the puppy to defecate and urinate on newspapers in the house, and then work on holding it until we get outside?**   Newspaper training is all right as a standby technique at night and when no one is at home, but during those times the animal should be confined on a newspaper-covered area anyway. It's a matter of convenience for the owner more than a training method, unless you live in a high-rise apartment and expect the dog to use the newspapers forever. Even then, newspaper training may be more trouble than it's worth; if you ever have to move, you'll face the difficult task of retraining the dog. That's why, even if you *do* use newspapers to train your dog, you should always combine the technique with training for elimination outdoors. The only exception would be the case of a very young pup if the weather is extremely cold or the ground is covered with thick snow. Using newspapers should be no more than supplemental training, good for two or three weeks. Take the papers away gradually until none are left. By the time the dog is twelve weeks old, he should be at the stage when he'll only eliminate outside; otherwise he'll become confused about where you want him to relieve himself.

**61. What should I do if I come home and see that my pup has eliminated in the house? She might have done it earlier, but is it okay to punish her when I discover the mess?**   Animals really don't understand this kind of punishment technique, and it does very little to correct their behavior. An animal doesn't remember when she's done something wrong in the house. You may *think* that a pup looks guilty when you discover her mischief, but what she's reacting to is your response. What you're going to have to do is reduce the chances of the pup's misbehaving. In other words, if the pup is eliminating in the house, you're going to have to make sure she's confined. The best time to actually discipline a pup is when you catch her in the act.

**62. My puppy is starting to chew constantly on furniture, shoes, just about everything. What can I do?**   Chewing is very natural behavior for a puppy, but it can get out of hand when the pup is left alone for long periods of time. To curb this habit, find a substance that has an unpleasant taste (for example, a commerical product that's also used to stop children from sucking their thumbs) and pass it lightly on the object the pup has been chewing. At the same time, douse a cotton ball with the substance and put it in the dog's mouth. Naturally, he'll spit it out—and when he does, praise him highly. Repeat this two or three times a day for about a week. As the dog begins to associate the unpleasant taste with the object, he'll stop chewing on it.

The most important thing to remember when you're dealing with this kind of problem is that you shouldn't leave the puppy *alone* in the house to chew on whatever he finds. Otherwise, you'll have to coat everything from the rugs to the sofa and the woodwork, and that will defeat the purpose of the whole exercise. Also give some thought to the toys you give your dog to chew on. You really shouldn't have more than two or three chew toys. A lot of people make the mistake of buying too many toys. The problem is that having *so many* toys means the dog doesn't discriminate between what he can and can't chew on. If he has two or three toys, he *knows* those are the only things he can chew on.

**63. *Our puppy isn't eating right, but he's begging at the table. How can we break him of this habit?*** Don't give in when he comes looking for handouts from the table. This is a bad habit to encourage. Instead, feed the dog *before* you eat. Let his food stay out for about two hours at the most, and if he hasn't eaten it by then, throw it away. If he gets nothing from you at the table, and sees his own food disappearing from neglect, he'll soon learn when and where he's supposed to eat.

**64. *How do I stop my pup from jumping up to greet me?*** When your pup jumps on you—or anyone else—make sure that he isn't petted; force him to get down on all fours in a sitting position before he's greeted or petted. It may look a bit odd, but when you come home, get down to the dog's level and pet him and greet him there. That way he'll learn to greet *you* from a sitting position. If this doesn't work, keep a leash attached to the dog's collar. When people come to the door, step on the leash so that when he gets up he's abruptly forced to sit down and keep *on* sitting. If *this* doesn't work, you might even have to resort to firmer action, such as putting your knee in his chest. You could also try stamping your foot or making a loud noise when the dog jumps up. Don't get discouraged if this kind of training takes longer than you expected—you may have to make a concerted effort for two or three weeks before you can start to control this kind of behavior.

**65. *We have a puppy that likes to bite. Although he doesn't do a lot of damage now, could this develop into a problem in the future?*** Indeed it could. Puppies use this playful nipping to establish dominance—when two pups play, they often bite each other lightly as they wrestle around. It's their way of working out social status. When it's applied to people, nipping should be promptly discouraged. Otherwise, the dog will keep this up and use it to try to dominate *you* by biting when he doesn't want to do something. In your relationship with the dog *you* should always be the dominant one. The dog should never modify *your* behavior.

To break a puppy of nipping, hold his snout shut with one hand, pick him up by the scruff of the neck with the other hand, and give him an authoritative shake, saying "No!" at the same time. Remember that you don't want to hurt the pup; just give him a clear message. Then put him down and play some more. If the puppy nips you again, repeat the punishment. If the pup *doesn't* nip your hand, praise and pet him. If he reverts to nipping later on, run through the whole sequence again (420).

*66. How early can you start teaching a puppy tricks, and what are the easiest ones to begin with?*   Don't expect a puppy to learn *anything* extra until she's gotten beyond basic housebreaking and the other fundamental training she needs. After your dog is three months old, her attention span should be long enough to make teaching her worth the effort. Be persistent and repetitive, and reward the dog for the right behavior. With some patience, you should have no trouble teaching the dog to sit, shake hands, roll over, speak, and fetch. Don't expect too much at first because a three-month-old dog has a hard time concentrating for very long; but by the time the dog is six to nine months old, she should be proficient at these tricks.

Use voice and hand signals when you're training the dog, but keep them as simple as possible. The animal can't follow a long, complicated gesture easily. Also, if you see the dog doing what you're trying to teach her—sitting, for example —then go over and say the command to her, and reinforce the command with petting. This may sound silly, but it will help the dog to connect the action with the instruction. Don't keep making the signal and saying the command when the dog is *not* doing what you want her to. Otherwise, they won't mean anything.

*67. How useful is professional training, and how early should it begin?*   It's very beneficial for all dogs to have some kind of formal training when they're around six months old. This can be a thorough obedience course with a professional trainer or just a group class with owners, dogs, and an instructor. In either case, the training procedures will give you a basis for working with your dog throughout his lifetime, even if the lessons are just fundamentals learned in a novice class. For more specific problems, such as car chasing or excessive aggression, a good trainer can be more valuable. Ask your veterinarian, breeder, or groomer for recommendation.

*68. How can I get my puppy used to riding in a car so he won't get sick every time we go somewhere?*   Start with short trips. Don't take the pup with you when it's hot or right after he's eaten; this could upset his stomach (169).

## Feeding

*69. Which of the three main types of dog food—canned, dry, and semi-moist patties—is best for my dog?*   In general, all three are nutritionally complete, but they have different qualities that should be considered when you're planning your dog's diet. Canned food is the least processed of the three, usually the lowest in protein, and soft in consistency. It's softness is its main drawback because it doesn't cleanse the dog's mouth as he eats. If you want to feed your dog canned food, it's a good idea to mix it with some dry food. Dry dog food is milled, the way a lot of cattle feed is produced. It generally has a more varied composition than canned food; it's made of grain pellets or even fish. The big advantage with dry food is its abrasive, cleansing action on the dog's teeth and mouth. Considering both the cost of dog food and its effect on your dog's health, I think a mixture of dry food and canned food is the best. The semi-moist dog-food patties are also nutritionally complete, and they usually provide more protein than canned food. However, they're highly processed, and they contain a lot of sugar. Semi-moist foods generally get their consistency from the addition of sucrose (corn syrup), which is bad for a dog's teeth. If the dog won't eat dry or canned food, semi-moist food is acceptable—mixed, if possible, with some dry food or at least a dog biscuit after the meal. Despite its limitations, it's better to feed your dog semi-moist food than it is to give him table scraps.

*70. How much protein does a dog need?*   A twenty-pound adult dog needs between 24 and 34 grams of usable protein each day, and puppies, pregnant dogs, and lactating females need about twice that amount. A can of dog food usually contains between 20 and 25 grams of usable protein. Some forms of protein aren't assimilated by the animal's digestive system, and they have no real food value. On the other hand, combinations of some foods provide more usable protein than the foods produce individually. For instance, if a dog is fed a cup and a half of brown rice at one meal and a half cup of beans at another, he would get a total of 20 grams of protein, but when the two foods are combined, they interact in the digestive system to provide 9 more grams of protein. Some other combinations that give bonus proteins are: rolled oats and milk; cornmeal, tofu (bean curd), and milk; and oats, eggs brewer's yeast, and milk. Remember too that the protein in one cup of milk is the same as that in one-third of a cup of powdered milk or half a cup of cottage cheese, both of which are much easier for a dog to digest than raw milk (36). Another factor to keep in mind is that some sources of protein are cleaner than others; in other words, the dog's kidneys don't have to work as hard to purify the animal's system after eating them. Eggs, poultry, fish, tofu, rice, and beans are more wholesome in this respect than beef, pork, or other sources of red meat. This can be crucial to a dog that has kidney disease (637).

*71. Is there some alternative to buying commercial dog food?*   Yes. You can make your own dog food, or you may be able to buy food wholesale from a feed mill in your area (72). To make your own, buy organ meat from the butcher—kidneys, liver, etc. Chop up the meat and boil it, then mix it with rice and cooked vegetables such as string beans or peas. If your dog will eat fish, this is also a good protein source, and so are eggs. Give a small dog two eggs a week, four to six for a medium-sized dog, and ten eggs a week will do for jumbo dogs (80). For pregnant dogs and pups, low-fat or dry milk should be sprinkled on the food for a boost in calcium (364). The meat should make up no more than forty percent of the dog's meal, with the other sixty percent divided evenly between vegetables and starch. Be sure to add a dog biscuit or an occasional meal of dry dog food to keep the dog's teeth clean.

*72. What's the best way to buy dog food in bulk quantities?*   If there's a mill in your area where cattle feed is made, it may be possible to buy bulk quantities of soy or cornmeal pellets, wheat-germ meal, or fish meal at a substantial savings. Some mills even make dog food and sell it wholesale. Whatever kind you decide to get, you'll want a small pellet size. It may be necessary to buy the food in 200-pound lots, so you might want to get together with some other dog owners and split up the load and the cost. To gauge how much you'll need, remember that a dog weighing 65 or 70 pounds will eat about 25 pounds of dog food in a month, or more.

*73. Can't dogs get along fine on an all-meat diet?*   No. Meat is deficient in some nutrients, vitamins, and minerals that are necessary for good health. If you plan to add meat to your dog's regular food, it should not be more than 40% of the meal.

*74. Is it all right for a dog to eat raw meat?*  Some health problems *can* arise from eating raw meat—trichinosis, for example. To avoid this, any meat you feed your dog should be cooked at least a little bit. To prepare the meat, boil it for about ten minutes.

*75. Isn't it true that dogs have an amazingly powerful stomach with digestive juices that can take care of just about anything?*  No. Dogs can only comfortably digest a small range of foods. Their diet is limited by their inability to chew, a predigestion process enjoyed by humans, as well as the fact that they have more simple digestive enzymes. Dogs have a lot of trouble with spicy foods, fruits, and raw vegetables.

*76. If dogs have such sensitive digestive systems, why don't they have a more discerning sense of smell and taste?*  Dogs are by nature scavengers, and many have become garbage hounds that will eat anything.

*77. Is is possible to keep a healthy dog on a vegetarian diet?*  Certainly. After all, the main ingredient in many dry dog foods is soybean or cornmeal protein. Eggs and powdered or low-fat milk are also good sources of protein. If you're going to add vegetables to these protein sources, they'll have to be cooked and bland so the dog can digest them properly (70). However, a dog *does* sometimes need a little animal fat to maintain a healthy coat (109).

*78. What kind of vegetables can I feed my dog?*  Certain vegetables are all right, as long as they're cooked and aren't strongly spiced. Beans (lima beans, string beans, peas) are an excellent source of protein. Well-cooked carrots and potatoes, combined with rice, are also good for bulk. Broccoli and cauliflower are good too. Avoid foods that are high in acid, such as tomatoes, peppers, eggplant, lettuce, and other raw greens. All of the vegetables you feed your dog have to be cooked. Unless you intend to maintain the dog on a complete and balanced vegetarian diet, it's best not to make vegetables more than about a quarter of the animal's total diet. And when you do this, remember to cut down the ration of regular food so that you don't over-feed the dog.

*79. Does the ash content of dog food affect an animal's health?*  High amounts of ash are suspected of causing urinary problems in cats, but there's no evidence that ash content has any effect on dogs. A possible relationship between ash content and bladder stones in dogs has been investigated, but no conclusive link has been found.

*80. Does raw egg white cause dietary problems for dogs?*  No. In cats, raw egg whites destroy certain vitamins, but this isn't the case with dogs.

*81. How important are vitamin supplements?*  It's best to give vitamin supplements *only* under the guidance of your vet. Otherwise, you can be wasting your money or even creating health problems for your dog. Once you've gotten the approval of your vet, extra vitamins *can* be helpful in several ways. Vitamins A, D, and E are good for the dog's coat and skin, and vitamin E also has some beneficial effects in relation to arthritis. Vitamin C builds the dog's immunity to various ailments and is good for the animal's bones. Puppies usually need some kind of supplement, especially for the B vitamins; these can be obtained in a multiple vitamin combination.

*82. Why are breeders so strongly in favor of vitamin C supplements?*   At this stage, it's almost like a health food fad. There's been some inconclusive evidence showing that large amounts of vitamin C may prevent hip dysplasia (601). Some reports say it can help if it's given to the bitch before whelping and to the pups afterward, but other reports dispute this. Vitamin C is water soluble, and, except in rare instances, it passes out of the body without causing any problems—so this practice doesn't hurt, even if it hasn't yet been proven effective. However, this vitamin theory doesn't take into account the genetic history of the individual dog, which may carry a tendency toward hip dysplasia. Probably the best insurance against hip dysplasia is simply not to breed a dog that has a history of this disease (343). However, if you want to try vitamin C, there's no harm in it. A pregnant dog with a family history of hip dysplasia should receive a gram a day of crystalline vitamin C (sodium ascorbic crystals). Puppies three to six months old take 500 milligrams per day; once they weigh eighty pounds or more, this can be increased gradually to one gram.

*83. Should I give my dog bones?*   Yes, but you should take some precautions because bones can cause problems. Bones can splinter and cause internal damage by perforating the esophagus, the stomach, or the small intestine, or by causing fecal impactions. *Never* give your dog poultry bones of any kind; they're thin and hollow, and they break up into sharp, dangerous slivers. Give a dog something really tough that he can gnaw on without making much headway. Watch his progress, and when he starts to break it open and splinter it, take it away and give him a new one.

*84. Is it true that garlic added to a dog's food helps keep off fleas and also guards against internal parasites?*   I know of no conclusive, scientific evidence about this, one way or the other—but some people swear by it, and since it can't hurt it might be worth a try. One clove mashed up in the dog's food every day should be plenty for the average dog; less for smaller ones. Brewer's yeast has also been shown to be helpful in warding off fleas (556).

*85. I've heard that alcohol can be good for dogs. Is that true?*   It *is* true—in moderation. Half a bottle of beer is about enough for an average-sized dog, but remember that beer is very fattening. If your dog has a weight problem, keep him on the wagon. Brandy is good for a dog with a cough or a cold. About eight drops mixed with a tablespoon of water will make him more comfortable.

*86. What can I do about my dog's flatulence?*   Have your dog checked for worms. If there's no problem, a diet change is necessary. The dog may be getting too many raw vegetables and fruits, or too much poorly processed commercial food that's partially indigestible. This sometimes happens when a dog eats a lot of dried food (especially those that contain large amounts of soybeans and cornmeal). Try cutting back on the dry food and substitute some canned food; this should help quite a bit. You could also give the dog bland homecooked food such as boiled chicken and rice.

*87. Is it true that some dogs will eat as much as you put before them, without limit, to the point of death?*   No. That's an exaggeration. However, some dogs will eat to the point of making themselves seriously ill. This is a carry-over from their days in the wild. Dogs, like present-day wolves, once fed on a large meal every two or three days, stuffing themselves while food was available and then going off to sleep and digest until hunger moved them to begin hunting again. Given the chance, larger dogs will still behave the same way, eating beyond their hunger drive.

**88. *Can gulping down a bowl of food be a danger to a dog's health?*** Dogs of German-shepherd size or larger can develop a condition called gastric torsion complex, or bloat, which can be fatal if it isn't treated quickly. Bloat occurs when the dog rapidly eats a bowl of dry food, then exercises or drinks a lot of water right afterward. This causes the stomach to swell up with gas and twist so that the gas can't escape. The stomach can get very large, and if it's not decompressed surgically the dog can die from shock. We don't know why the stomach twists, but this sealing action prevents the use of a stomach tube to relieve the pressure.

**89. *How can "bloat" be prevented?*** Mix canned food with the dog's dry food. Try dividing a meal into two, three, or even four portions, and feeding them to the dog over the course of the day, with at least half an hour between feedings. Don't let the dog exercise for an hour after eating, and don't let him drink a lot of water right after eating. You can also prevent bloat by looking for dry food that's labelled "non-expandable." Many dry dog foods are puffed up with air in the processing, and these are the ones you want to avoid if you have a large dog that eats only dry food.

**90. *Should you feed a very active dog more than one that gets very little exercise?*** Yes. A working dog, such as a hunting hound or a dog that jogs with you regularly, will need more food on days when she's putting out extra energy. A working dog should have her meals increased by 30 or 40%. Feed the dog twice—once in the morning, before the day's activities begin, and again in the evening. The first meal should be lighter than the dog's supper, but it's important that the animal have *something* to eat before beginning a work-out.

**91. *What can I feed an underweight dog to help her gain weight?*** First, make sure the dog is actually underweight. Some dogs look thin, but may be within the normal range of weight for their breed and be perfectly healthy. Have the dog's condition evaluated by your veterinarian if there's any doubt. If you've found a stray or you have a dog that's been ill for a long time and has suffered from loss of appetite, bulk up her diet with more carbohydrates—rice, bread, or spaghetti. If the dog was a stray, she may be quite malnourished, so give her twenty-five percent more food than a normal serving, with a double portion of vitamin and mineral supplements.

**92. *Do dogs develop health problems from cholesterol the way people do?*** Dogs are lucky in that they don't suffer from hardening of the arteries, but they *do* have some problems that are related to fatty foods. Pancreatitis, an inflamed gastro-intestinal tract, comes from eating too many table scraps or too much garbage. For smaller dogs, there's a danger of getting huge fat deposits in the liver that impair its ability to function. And, of course, dogs can become overweight.

**93. *How serious a problem is obesity for a dog?*** A badly overweight dog can develop a lot of troubles—liver disease, pancreatitis (92), back troubles, and heart disease. The dog tends to become overheated more quickly, so heat stroke is a greater danger. An overweight dog also finds it harder to breathe.

**94. *Is it okay to put a dog on a starvation diet?*** If your dog is very fat, don't immediately put her on a starvation diet. This could damage the animal's health. Instead, gradually cut back the amount of food the dog normally gets, by about 20 percent each day, until you reach a proper level for weight loss (95).

**95. *We have a fat dog. How do we start taking off all that extra weight?*** It takes discipline, but it *can* be done. There are commercial diets for dogs that make it fairly easy to adjust the amount of calories he's getting. You just have to adhere to them strictly—no table scraps and no treats. Before starting a diet, the dog should have a full physical examination; there may be a need for vitamin supplements, or there may be other medical considerations to keep in mind. Once the dog has been checked, figure out how much you want him to lose; ask your vet if you aren't sure. Suppose you want the dog to go from 75 pounds to 60. You'll have to calculate how much a 60-pound dog should eat, then cut this back another 20%. You can make up the 20% cut with low-calorie bulk such as cottage cheese or green beans. These will fill the dog up and keep him from being constantly hungry. Once he gets close to the desired weight—60 pounds in our example—then bring the ration of diet mix up to a 60-pound dog's level. Keep a record of the dog's progress by weighing him weekly.

**96. *Should I combine a diet with an exercise program?*** Ask your vet about this because it depends on the age and physical condition of the dog. However, you can look forward to seeing the dog become more active as the diet takes effect. When a dog is fat, his instinctive after-meal lethargy becomes a cycle of eating and lying around. By breaking this cycle, you can expect a much more lively dog.

**97. *I've tried putting my dog on a commercial diet program, but she doesn't want to eat it. Should I go back to her old food or hold out until hunger forces her to eat?*** A healthy, small dog can go for about three days without eating and suffer no adverse effects, and large dogs can safely go without food for five days, so don't give in immediately if she turns up her nose at the diet food. However, if she absolutely refuses to eat it, there *is* an alternative. If the dog regularly eats a can of dog food, you can cut this amount to three quarters. If the dog is *still* very hungry and this just isn't enough food, then give her half a can of dog food and half a portion made up of low-calorie bulk foods such as cottage cheese or green beans. If the dog has been on a long hunger strike because she doesn't like the diet mix you bought, there's no sense in blowing her eating capacity back up again with bulk additives. Just give her a reduced portion of her regular food. Her stomach will have grown smaller while she wasn't eating, and she'll probably never notice the difference.

**98. *What can I do about a picky eater that walks away from regular dog food and pesters me for table food?*** Once a dog develops a taste for scraps, it's hard to break this habit. Rather than eat dry food, and even some canned foods, some of these dogs will actually starve to the point of becoming seriously malnourished. This is a common problem, and one that can do a lot of damage to a dog's health. All too often, I see over-indulged, spoiled dogs who have terrible teeth and gum decay because they never eat dry food. To control this bad habit, start with a confrontation. Offer the dog *dog* food, and if that's not good enough, let him go hungry for a day or so. Of course, some dogs will *never* give in, and may hold out until they're dangerously undernourished—so if your dog won't give in after three days, buy some organ meat from the butcher (liver, kidney, something cheap), then cook it up with some rice for bulk, and add a little dry dog food. Do this for several days, each day increasing the amount of dry food and cutting back on the rice and meat. You may not be able to use this ploy to totally change the dog's diet, but you can probably get the little gourmet to eat half and half without a lot of trouble.

**99. *I used to give my dog a piece of candy when I came home from work, and now that I've retired he wants one every ten minutes. How can I stop this constant begging?*** If your dog is used to getting a snack every time he comes begging, switch him over to dog biscuits at first—they're low in calories. Break off pieces of them, gradually reducing the amount as the days go by. Occasionally give the dog a treat when he's *not* begging so that he begins to lose the association between whining and receiving a treat. Cut out the treats slowly so that the dog doesn't feel suddenly deprived, but do it *before* you have the added problem of putting a fat dog on a diet.

## Grooming

**100. *How often should I brush my dog?*** For the average dog, one that isn't shedding too much or having skin problems, twice a week is usually enough. Remember, though, that the need for brushing depends on the kind of coat the dog has. A longhaired dog, such as a sheepdog or a Lhasa apso, needs about 15 minutes of daily brushing and a thorough going-over, which can take as long as an hour, once a week. These dogs should also be taken to a professional groomer twice a year to be clipped. A shorthaired dog, such as a weimaraner or a Labrador retriever, needs only about a ten-minute grooming session twice a week, while dogs with moderately long hair, such as collies or golden retrievers, can get along being groomed three times a week for about fifteen minutes at a time. Poodles are a special case where grooming is concerned because they don't shed. They need to be groomed three times a week, and they require a professional clipping job at least twice a year.

**101. *What kind of grooming tools will I need for my dog?*** Use a wire brush with stiff bristles on a longhaired dog; this will help break up matted hair and brush out shedding fur. For small, woolly dogs you'll need to use a wire brush, followed by a wide-toothed comb to get out any knots. A soft- to medium-bristled brush is best for

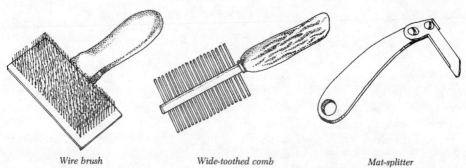

Wire brush          Wide-toothed comb          Mat-splitter

shorthaired dogs because it will help eliminate dander flakes as well as unwanted hair. For dogs that have kinky hair with a tendency to form mats, there's a very useful tool called a mat and tangle splitter. This is a simple razor blade with a protective point that can't cut the dog; it's good for breaking down mats so they can be trimmed or brushed out. Specially made manual or electric clippers are also useful.

*102. Is there any special way you should brush a dog?*   Just follow the direction of the dog's coat and make the strokes long, from front to back.

*103. Why do dogs shed?*   A dog sheds in the fall to replace a thin summer coat with a thicker winter fur, and again in the spring to thin out the winter coat in preparation for the warmer days ahead. This loss of hair is guided by the length of the day, the amount of light the dog experiences. When the days get shorter, the dog starts to shed for his winter coat, and when the daylight reaches a longer threshold the animal begins to prepare for summer. Because of this, a lot of dogs that are kept inside the house—and are exposed to artificial light at night—shed more than they naturally would, or even shed all year round.

*104. Can the amount of shedding be reduced somehow? Can I brush out all the loose hair at once?*   Brushing can help minimize the mess, but you'll never be able to brush out all the shedding hair. The best way to reduce shedding is to lubricate the dog's skin and coat by adding polyunsaturated fat to the animal's diet (106). You can also improve the condition of the dog's coat by giving him vitamin A, D, and E supplements. Check with your vet for the proper dosage for your dog.

*105. How should a healthy dog's coat look?*   The fur should be fairly glossy, with little or no flakes from the skin. There will always be *some* shedding, but this should not be excessive. The appearance of a dog's coat changes over the years, but this is greatly influenced by the food the dog eats. A well-maintained coat requires a lot of protein and all the proper vitamins (70, 81).

*106. Do dogs get dandruff? How is it treated?*   Dogs get a skin disease called seborrhea (530) that shows up in different ways, and one of them is dandruff-like flaking and dry skin. If you see this on your dog, it's best to have him examined by your veterinarian because the condition could be a symptom of an internal metabolic problem. If it's simple seborrhea, there are specific dog dandruff shampoos available, or you can use any mild, coal-tar human dandruff shampoo (116). The dog's diet should also be supplemented with brewer's yeast and polyunsaturated oil (wheatgerm oil, corn oil, or sunflower-seed oil). The daily dose for both should be one tablespoon for every 20 pounds of the dog's weight. Combine this with supplements of vitamins A, E, and D at dosages prescribed by your vet, who can also supply you with a mixture of oils and vitamins if you don't want to buy them separately.

*107. My Irish setter has a dull, flaky coat. Is this caused by a dietary deficiency?*   Possibly. However, Irish setters and golden retrievers often have underactive thyroid glands, and this condition shows up on their coats in cycles of flaking and dullness. If your dog is getting plenty of the proper food and vitamins, and sufficient oils and dietary fats, the thyroid could be the source of the trouble. The condition can be treated with synthetic thyroid hormones.

*108. What dietary supplements does a dog with dry skin problems need?*   Vitamins A, D, and E will help, and you can also add cod liver oil or vegetable oil to the dog's diet. One teaspoon of cod liver oil daily for every ten pounds of dog weight is enough; double that if you're using vegetable oil. Even with these supplements, the dog will also need some animal fat every day (109).

*109. Should I give my dog a pat of butter every day to improve his coat?* No. Because it's a dairy product, butter doesn't metabolize very well in dogs. A dog needs *animal* fat—bacon drippings or a little bit of grease or fatty meat. The rule of thumb for the daily dosage is one teaspoon for every twenty pounds of the dog's weight.

*110. Is it safe to cut off matted lumps of hair at home?* Yes, but don't use scissors— this is a frequent cause of injuries. A dog's skin is very loose, and when you're using scissors you can often pick up the skin along with a clump of matted hair and accidentally inflict a nasty cut. It's much safer to use a manual or electric clippers.

*111. What's the best way to clean tar, paint, and chewing gum out of a dog's coat?* The easiest way to get rid of chewing gum is to clip it out of the dog's coat. (A little ice applied to the gum can reduce the stickiness and make it easier to work with.) This shouldn't be a very large area, and the fur will grow back quickly. The same method should work for paint. Don't use paint thinners or kerosene because it could harm the animal's skin, and there's a good chance the dog will lick some off and swallow it. Tar is a mess that can also be removed by clipping—but if there's too much to be easily trimmed you can try removing it with petroleum jelly. This may take a while, but it's the safest way of getting tar off the dog. It's important to get the tar off the dog before he has a chance to chew at it because tar is toxic. Just rub the jelly into the tar spot; it will mix with the tar and thin it out. If you keep applying the jelly and rubbing it off with a rag, the dog's coat should eventually come clean.

*112. Is it a good idea to clip a longhaired dog's coat for the summer?* Yes. This is a good idea for *any* woolly, longhaired dog. Just be sure to leave at least three to four inches of fur—the hair serves as protection from the sun, and it can actually insulate the animal from excessive heat. A dog's fur grows back in three or four months, so one clipping will probably last for a whole summer.

*113. Is it safe to trim the hair out of a dog's eyes.?* Yes. If the hair is so long and thick that the dog can't see well, go ahead and trim it back—the dog is in no danger. Many people believe that this hair protects a dog's eyes from the light, and that her eyes may be damaged or blinded if the hair is trimmed. This just isn't true. The hair has nothing to do with the light sensitivity of the dog's eyes.

*114. How should I select a professional groomer?* Just ask your veterinarian to recommend one, or ask friends who have the same type of dog that you have. Breeders will also be able to give you the names of reputable groomers. The most important thing to keep in mind when you're dealing with groomers is the fact that they're only permitted to give a dog tranquilizers under the supervision of a vet. If your dog is nervous and uncomfortable when he's being groomed, talk to your vet about prescribing a tranquilizer and *then* consult with the groomer. Never patronize a groomer who uses tranquilizers on your dog and doesn't discuss this with you first.

*115. How often should I bathe my dog?* If a dog spends a lot of time outside she should get a bath once a week during warm weather. Any normal, healthy dog should be bathed about once a month in the summer, but this is something you can judge by the dog's appearance and smell. In the winter, the dog may need to be bathed only once, or not at all. Small, short-coated breeds sometimes have very little odor, and they may require minimal bathing year-round.

*116. What's the best way to bathe a dog?*   First, put a little petroleum jelly over the dog's eyebrows (and on a male dog's scrotum) to protect them from soap burns. If you'll be bathing the dog inside, run a couple of inches of lukewarm water into the tub *before* you put the dog in it so that he won't be startled by the noise. Get the dog thoroughly wet—you can use a sponge to slop water over him—and then apply the soap. Use special dog shampoo or baby shampoo; anything stronger will dry out the dog's coat. If you're using a medicated or flea-and-tick shampoo, leave it on for five minutes before rinsing; otherwise you can just clean the dog up after he's been lathered. Rinse him thoroughly with running water or water dipped up with a pan or cup. A cream rinse can also be applied to a dog with dry skin problems. Make sure you rinse off *all* the shampoo because any residue will dry and stick to your dog's skin, and he'll begin scratching at it. Once you've rinsed the dog thoroughly, dry him off with a towel (or a hand-held dryer if the noise and the air flow don't bother him). Just to be sure that he doesn't catch cold, it's a good idea to keep your dog inside for a few hours until you're sure he's thoroughly dry. In the summertime, when there's little danger of his catching cold, the whole bathing process can be done outside. Then you can use a hose to bathe your dog, or you can try a plastic baby swimming pool for a small dog that may not like being squirted.

*117. How useful is a dry bath?*   Powder baths are no substitute for the real thing. If the weather is very cold and you think a wet bath could be dangerous, then go ahead with a dry bath. If you don't have a longhaired dog, you can try using cornmeal instead of the commercial products. Just powder it on and brush it out thoroughly.

*118. What do you recommend for removing skunk scent from a dog?*   Start with a long, thorough scrubbing in the bathtub. Then slop a lot of tomato juice all over the dog's coat. Let this stay on for ten or fifteen minutes, and then rinse off. Bathe again, douse again, and continue until the smell is gone or at least tolerable.

## Caring for Nails, Ears, and Teeth

*119. What age should my dog be when I start trimming her nails.?*   Of all the routine care that dogs must undergo, nail clipping is what they hate most. You can make this chore easier if you start early (48). It's also medically important to begin trimming the dog's nails from the time it's a puppy (120).

*120. Are there medical reasons for trimming a dog's nails?*   Nothing serious, but there *are* four basic problems that can occur if a dog's nails aren't cared for. (1) If the nails aren't cut from an early age, the vein grows down inside the claw as the pup matures, making it necessary to keep the claw long from then on. (2) The dog's dew claws—the small, rudimentary toes on the inside of the dog's leg—can curl around and grow back into the dog's flesh if they aren't trimmed. (3) Small dogs sometimes develop a problem as they get older if their claws aren't properly trimmed—the toes begin to spread apart, and walking becomes difficult. This happens most often in dogs that don't support much weight and rarely walk on concrete. (4) Long nails can sometimes snag and this can damage the dog's foot.

**121. How often do I have to trim my dog's nails?** If the dog walks a lot on concrete, the nails are usually filed down enough just by daily activities. Dogs that spend most of their time indoors or on grass need their nails trimmed when they begin to hook and sharpen. For most dogs, this will be about once a month. Remember, though, that the nails can't be trimmed back so short and blunt that they won't be felt when the dog jumps up. When the nails are beginning to point and curve, then it's time for a trim.

**122. What kind of clippers should I use to trim my dog's nails?** Unless you have a very small dog, you won't be able to use human nail clippers because a dog's claws are very thick. A specially made set of nail clippers is a good investment, and one 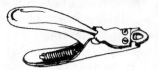 that you should buy as soon as you get a new dog. That way the pup will become accustomed to their use at an early age. The clippers make trimming a dog's nails as efficient as possible because the end of the claw sticks through so that you can see what you're cutting, but there's no sharp point that can cut the dog accidentally. These tools come in three different sizes, so get one that's right for your dog. Look for the kind that has a blade that can be removed and sharpened.

**123. Why are a dog's back nails almost always shorter than the ones in front?** When a dog starts to walk or run, he pushes off with his hindquarters. Because of the abrasive action, you may never have to trim your dog's back claws.

**124. I know a dog's nails can bleed. How much can I safely trim off?** If the nails are white, you have the advantage of being able to see where the blood is circulating—the blood vessels show up clearly as the red portion of the nail. Cut just a little bit in front of this area. If the nails are black, you won't have the blood mark as a guide, but there *is* something else that you can use as a 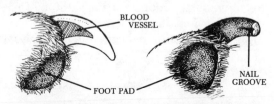 reference point. The dog's nails will have a slight groove where they split on the underside of the curve. If you cut just in *front* of this split, you should miss the vein.

**125. What should I do if I cut too far and the dog's nail starts to bleed?** This kind of injury looks much worse than it actually is because the dog's claw tends to bleed a great deal. The best treatment is to apply the kind of alum sulfate pencil that's used to stop bleeding in shaving cuts. If this isn't available, hold cold compresses to the foot for about ten minutes. Cold water on a clean rag or a wad of cotton will serve as a compress; hold it tightly to the bleeding surface, applying mild pressure.

**126. What are dew claws?** These dangling little growths on the inside of the legs are vestiges of a thumb. A dog has only four toes on each foot, with a dew claw located about two inches up the leg in a place where, eons ago, a thumb used to be. As the dog evolved, this digit ceased to be useful and withered to its present condition.

**127. Can dew claws be a problem?**   Normally there's nothing to worry about, provided the nail is kept trimmed along with the rest of the dog's nails—but if a dog has exceptionally loose, large dew claws, they might get snagged, especially the ones on the rear legs, where the dog doesn't pay as much attention to his steps. Breeders of large dogs generally have the dew claws cropped off when they dock the pup's tail (430). This habit may have some useful function for hunting dogs, but for many breeds it's purely a cosmetic operation.

**128. How can I protect my dog's feet from ice in the winter?**   Icy streets are rough on a dog's feet, but what's even worse is the rock salt that's spread on sidewalks to melt the ice. Salt gets caught in the dog's foot along with the ice, where it becomes partially frozen and causes painful irritations by literally rubbing salt into the wounds it creates. Put a little petroleum jelly on the dog's foot pads before going for a walk. When you return, wash the animal's feet and rub in a little skin lotion to soothe the foot pads and prevent the skin from cracking.

**129. Will my dog's feet be injured by too much contact with pavement?**   It's possible. Running for a long distance on hard pavement will tear up the foot pad, which is, after all, just a callus. Be specially mindful of this if your dog spends a lot of time on the grass—don't run the dog on cement until he's had a chance to get used to it.

**130. My dog's foot pads have little cracks in them. Is this an injury?**   Foot pads, like most calluses, get occasional cracks and fissures. This is nothing to worry about as long as the cracks don't extend all the way through the pad and you can't see the pink flesh underneath. *If* there is a deep break in the pad, it will need treatment because the dog has lost a natural barrier against infection. Wash the pad with an antiseptic solution and keep it bandaged until it's had a chance to heal (about a week, or even a little longer). Change the bandage every other day.

**131. How often should a dog's ears be cleaned?**   The shape of the ear is important here. Dogs with long, floppy ears (such as pointers, poodles, and beagles) should require cleaning about twice a month; and dogs with ears that stand up (such as German shepherds and Doberman pinschers) need even less attention—no more than once a month under normal conditions, if at all. This generally holds true no matter what the size of the dog. Dogs that have the flaking skin problem of sebborhea (106) will also have an accompanying waxy build-up in the ears that should be cleaned about once a week. This condition can be controlled but not cured, so it will require continual attention. A human ear wash will cut through the wax quite efficiently.

To tell if your dog's ears need cleaning, look for a slight waxy build-up and a mild, greasy odor that's noticeable, but not unpleasant. If the odor is foul, this is a sign of infection (134). If the ears look clean and have no waxy build-up or odor, just leave well enough alone. Probing around might only cause problems.

**132. What's the best way to clean a dog's ears?**   Use cotton dipped in mineral oil and your fingertip. If the ear is particularly clogged with wax, you can get a solution from the vet that will break up the deposit. After a couple of days of this treatment, the ears can then be cleaned with cotton and mineral oil. Cotton swabs are not recommended for cleaning a dog's ears because they can actually impact material further into the ear.

**133. Is there risk of damaging the dog's eardrum while cleaning the ear?** The structure of a dog's ear makes it almost impossible to break the eardrum, but if the dog has a bad infection there *is* a danger of impacting material in the bottom of the outer ear or pressing wax deposits against the eardrum. This is why you should always clean the dog's ears properly (132), being careful never to push any material more deeply into the ear canal.

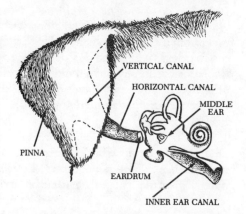

**134. How can I tell if my dog's ears are infected?** Normal ear wax for dogs is golden to light brown in color; anything darker is usually a sign of infection. In most cases, there's also a bad odor, and possibly a discharge of yellow or brown pus. The dog's behavior is also a clue. He may shake his head and scratch at one or both ears. When you notice this, take the dog in for a check-up. The shaking and scratching could be a sign of an infection or an infestation of ear mites, an extremely irritating parasite that's usually picked up from cats (566). Both need the attention of a vet, but for mild infections—and as a first aid measure until the dog can be taken to the vet—clean the ear (132) and then wipe on a mild antiseptic solution with a cotton ball. Apply the antiseptic every day for four or five days and clean the ear every third day. If the condition doesn't improve, have your dog examined by your vet.

**135. Are antibiotic preparations for humans useful in treating ear infections in dogs?** Despite any medical benefits they may have, these over-the-counter products generally are no help for ear infections because of their gel form. An ear infection needs air circulation to heal, and the waxy deposits already in the ear make this difficult enough without further cutting off the problem area with a cream or gel. Antibiotic powders are also ineffective because they don't penetrate far enough. Antibiotic ointments are available by prescription, and these are about the best.

**136. Is there any way to prevent ear infections?** Yes. Ear infections are frequently caused by an overgrowth of hair in the dog's ear that blocks drainage and air circulation. When the hair starts to become too thick, it needs to be plucked out. You can do this with your fingers, or you can use tweezers for a better grip. A dog with a lot of hair in her ears should have that hair plucked every month. This is mostly a problem for smaller dogs, particularly Lhasa apsos, poodles, and other breeds with thick, woolly coats. Don't pluck too much at one time because if there's any inflammation the plucking will make the infection worse.

**137. Why is it customary to clip some dog's ears and tails?** Originally there was a practical reason for this. The dogs were used in hunting and fighting, and these extremities were trimmed so that they wouldn't be targets for their opponents. Nowadays, this cropped appearance has become a standard for several breeds, carried on mostly because people expect it.

*138. Are there medical difficulties to watch out for in cropping a dog's ears and tail?* A dog's tail can be bobbed quite easily in the first week after birth. At that age the tail hasn't developed to the point where there's a significant bleeding problem, and no recovery time is required. Ear cropping, on the other hand, is done when the dog is eight weeks old, and it's a messy operation. The ears usually have to remain bandaged for a period of from two weeks to two months. There's a danger of infection after the ears have been cropped, and this is sometimes made worse by the dog's natural tendency to scratch his ears.

*139. Do dogs get cavities in their teeth?* In general they do not. Their teeth are mostly sharp and smooth, without the close, grinding surfaces and pockets that can trap food and cause decay in human teeth. Also, food just doesn't stay in a dog's mouth long enough to have much effect on the teeth—it's down too quickly for that.

*140. My dog's teeth build up tartar very quickly. What can I do about it?* Dry dog food and dog biscuits generally have an abrasive, cleansing effect on teeth, so a change in diet, substituting some dry food for canned food, will help. You can also give the dog a couple of dog biscuits about ten minutes after every meal.

*141. My dog has bad breath. What causes this, and how can I get rid of it?* This is usually caused by a tooth problem called periodontal disease that, in turn, is caused by years of tartar build-up along the gumline. It's especially common in dogs with malocclusion—their teeth don't meet properly, so there are certain areas where food residues can build up. When this happens, bacteria invade the dog's gums, giving rise to the offensive breath problem. Once this process begins, it won't go away completely, but it *can* be slowed down by having the dog's teeth cleaned and scaled by a veterinarian and then treating the dog with antibiotics to kill the bacteria. To reduce future bacteria build-up, brush the dog's teeth with toothpaste, baking soda, or peroxide gel, a human gum-care product that's available in drugstores. If a toothbrush is too stiff for the dog's mouth, use a gauze pad to clean the teeth.

## Dog Paraphernalia

*142. What's the best kind of collar for my dog?* A leather or nylon buckle collar is fine for a small dog. You can also use one on a larger dog that isn't being trained. Just make sure that the collar is large enough so that it doesn't fit too tightly around the dog's neck, but not *so* loose that it will slip off over the animal's head. The collar should hang a little bit loosely on the dog's neck. This type of collar will double for a training collar on small breeds, but for larger dogs most people use some kind of choker collar, provided the dog doesn't suffer from a collapsible trachea (521). Chokers come in three basic forms—nylon, chain, and angle-pronged chain. A nylon choker is usually most effective on smaller breeds because training these dogs doesn't require a great deal of leverage and pressure. A chain choker is necessary for bigger dogs. Whatever choker you need, get one that fits loosely around the dog's neck. Remember, it isn't the pressure of the choker that disciplines the dog as much as the surprise of its sudden constriction. If the collar is always a little bit tight around the dog's neck, the animal may not notice the extra tightness when you pull on the leash. An angle-pronged collar should only be used on a dog that's *very* large and is at least nine months old—and *only* after a chain collar has proven ineffective. This kind of collar is designed to apply a lot of pressure to the animal's neck without hurting it. Such a collar can be useful as a training tool, but only for a dog that has a sturdy neck.

*143. Do those broad collars with big spikes have any functional use?* Yes. The spikes protect the dog from bites to the neck—a dog's favorite target in a fight.

*144. Is there any advantage in outfitting a dog with a harness instead of a collar?* There *are* instances when a harness can be very useful. For a dog with a weak trachea, a harness can prevent a lot of choking and gagging (521). A harness is also good for a dog that has a neck irritation from a flea collar or a choker chain.

*145. What kind of muzzle do you recommend?* A cage-type muzzle is good for garbage eaters, but if you want to keep a dog from biting the safest kind of muzzle is a cone-shaped one. The *least* secure is a leather muzzle that looks like a horse's bridle. It's the hardest to put on, and the least effective. Of course, you should *never* rely

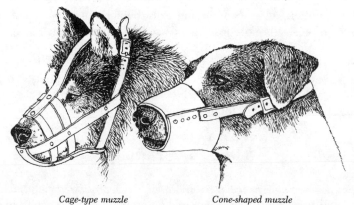

Cage-type muzzle          Cone-shaped muzzle

solely on a muzzle to protect people from your dog—it's not a substitute for training. But if you have a dog that bites, it's an excellent idea for everyone's benefit if you muzzle the animal before bringing him to the veterinarian's office. It makes working with a dog much easier and it allows for a more thorough examination.

*146. What should I look for when I'm buying a leash?* First, make sure you get a leash that's strong enough to restrain your dog. A chain leash usually isn't as strong as a sturdy leather or nylon leash; chain leashes are also heavier, tend to rust, and can pinch your hand. Make sure you get a leash that's long so that you can use it for training and double it up short for city walking. When you're training a dog, it's important that the leash be long so that you can put a lot of leverage into a yank on the choker collar; otherwise, the dog won't get the message (226).

**147. *Is a silent dog whistle a useful piece of equipment or just a novelty?*** A silent whistle can definitely be useful in training your dog. It's harder to use than hand signals or voice commands, but it has the advantage of greater range—and neighbors will appreciate its silence.

**148. *What kind of bowl should I buy for my dog?*** Of course, the size depends on the type of dog you have. As far as the *kind* of bowl goes, I'd recommend that you get a ceramic or stainless steel bowl instead of a plastic one because some dogs are allergic to plastic (527). It's also a good idea to know how much a bowl holds so you can gauge the amount of food the dog is getting. Actually, there's no reason that a formal "dog" bowl has to be used at all. Whether you use a shallow or a deep bowl is a matter of personal preference, as long as the dog is able to feed out of it and reach the bottom with no trouble. Remember, though, that it's easier to spill food out of a shallow bowl, and dogs aren't noted for their good table manners.

**149. *Should I buy my dog a bed?*** Most of the time I think this is unnecessary. Besides, if you get a bed for a puppy, he's likely to chew it up and defecate and urinate in it. An older dog can get used to a commercially made bed more easily, but the only real purpose I can see for one would be to keep an old, arthritic dog off a damp floor—and you can improvise something for a lot less money.

**150. *Does a dog really need a doghouse?*** This is generally a good idea if the dog spends a lot of time outside. Make sure you have one that's roomy. It should also be raised off the ground so that the floor doesn't get too cold in the winter; insulation also helps keep the temperature in the house safe and comfortable. A doghouse can also help prevent heat stroke when the sun is hot. Remember to clean and disinfect the doghouse regularly; about once a week is fine. Don't put a rug or any kind of cloth in the doghouse—this will only make cleaning harder and serve as a hideout for fleas.

**151. *I'm buying a small dog. Will I need a carrying case for her?*** Very small dogs often are nervous when they're being carried from one place to another, so the kind of carrying case that's used for cats can help them feel secure. However, before you spend this extra money make sure that the dog won't be sufficiently calmed just by being carried in your arms. Larger dogs that are being shipped or can't walk for some reason will need a cage. This can also be used in their training, and it can be a good investment (50).

**152. *Are dog sweaters useful?*** These are good for small breeds in extremely cold climates. They're also useful should the dog have to be clipped in the winter.

**153. *What about boots for dogs to protect their feet?*** These are all right, although most dogs won't tolerate them. And it's also possible to *over*protect the dog to the point where the foot pads become too soft, leaving the foot open to greater injury when cold weather ends and the dog is barefoot again.

*154. What's the best kind of toy for my dog?*  The most sensible guide in choosing toys is: the tougher they are, the better they are. A hard rubber ball is one of the best things you can buy. It's chewy, bouncy, and difficult to shred and swallow (62).

*155. Is it all right to give my dog one of those hollow rubber toys with a squeaker inside?*  I think they're dangerous. These toys are flimsy and a dog can rip one up in no time. After that, it's easy to swallow pieces of rubber and metal, and the dog could choke or damage his digestive tract. Find your dog a more rugged toy.

*156. I've heard that rawhide toys are bad for dogs. Is this true?*  It depends on the toy and the size of the dog. It's good to give a dog something to chew on, and for this a rawhide toy is hard to beat. The potential problem arises when the dog starts to swallow the pieces. Rawhide fibers aren't digestible, although they will pass through the animal's system—a little bit of rawhide is acceptable, but a lot can really upset the dog's digestive system. The best solution is simply to avoid giving the dog anything she can chew up quickly; give her a toy that will take about a week to destroy. When she can rip off pieces without a lot of trouble, or when the toy gets too small, take it away and give her a new one.

*157. Are there any toys that I can make at home for my dog?*  Dogs are so destructive when they play with something that it's hard to find common household materials that are durable enough to make successful dog toys. I've seen puppies swallow whole socks; obviously, that isn't a good way to recycle worn-out clothing. In addition, you don't want to get the dog used to playing with clothes or old shoes because the animal will never be able to distinguish between a discard and your new pair of wing tips. Old tennis balls are all right, as long as the dog isn't too big. A large dog can shred a tennis ball in minutes and swallow parts of it—so if you see the ball being ripped up, take it right away. It may cost a little bit to buy a hard rubber ball from a pet shop, but it's still the best thing you can give a dog to play with.

## Exercise

*158. How much exercise does a dog really need, and how soon should I start some kind of regular schedule?*  You can begin a daily exercise routine when the dog is three months old. A mature dog—four months to ten years old—should be walked at least three times a day and allowed free exercise for thirty minutes or more a minimum of twice a week, no matter what the breed or size. Little dogs can get this exercise inside an apartment or home. It's also a good idea to do as much running and playing on grass as you can. Pavement can be very damaging to a dog's feet, especially with the kind of sprinting and stopping that go along with most play.

Don't overtax the dog. Watch to make sure she isn't getting too hot and tired, especially on a warm day. If you notice that the dog tires quickly from a routine that gave her no trouble before, take her to the veterinarian for a check-up—this can be an early sign of heart and lung trouble. When a dog passes the age of ten, start cutting back on the exercise, particularly if her breed is prone to hip problems (182). Finally, if you're running a male dog where there may be other dogs around, be sure to keep track of him. The temptation to roam and the opportunity to mate can turn the romp into a fight—or a litter of unwanted puppies.

**159. Is there any particular kind of exercise that's best for my dog?**  It's good to pick an exercise that's appropriate for your particular breed. For instance, a retriever loves to chase and fetch a ball or a stick, and a husky will enjoy pulling a sled in the winter or a small cart during warm weather. You can take traditional hunting dogs such as a weimaraner or a setter for a run through the woods, and if you live near water, retrievers and springer spaniels are particularly fond of swimming (132).

**160. Is it bad to exercise my dog right after he's been fed?**  Yes, but don't wait *too* long. After a big meal, a dog wants to lie down and digest for a long time, a habit that contributes quite a bit to obesity problems. Wait about an hour after a dog has eaten before trying any strenuous activity.

**161. Is there anything I should watch out for when I let my dog go swimming?**  Don't take your dog swimming where the banks are high and the animal can't easily crawl out or find the bottom. A gradually rising bottom, such as that found at a beach, is ideal. However, be careful if you take your dog to the ocean because she could panic if the surf is strong or if she swims out over her head—and you might have to do some quick lifesaving. Play with your dog in the shallow surf, but call her back if she starts to swim out where the water is over her head.

**162. Is it all right to jog with my dog?**  Yes, but there are some important considerations to take beforehand, especially if you'll be running long distances. Make sure the dog is in good health. He should have been checked in the last year by your veterinarian, and there should be no evidence of heartworms, arthritis, or hip dysplasia. And before you start your run, remember that the dog needs to warm up as much as you do—give him some preliminary exercise by letting him retrieve a stick or ball. Start running slowly, and increase the distance covered gradually. A medium-sized dog should eventually have no difficulty pacing you for five or ten miles.

**163. Is it possible to run the dog too far?**  Yes. Remember that dogs are notorious for overtaxing themselves. If you let them, they'll enthusiastically play and run until they drop with exhaustion. If you see that the dog is beginning to pant heavily, stop running and find a cool place to rest. Also keep in mind the fact that the dog's tolerance for heat is low. It may be best to run alone on a hot day or cut the run short, particularly if your dog has long hair (462). If at any time the dog comes up lame don't continue to run him because this can make the problem worse. If the limp persists, take the dog to your vet (475).

**164. What about the dog's feet? Will they be hurt by a long run?**  Yes. Watch out for broken glass, and always check the dog's paws after a run. If they're cut or scraped, don't run her again until they heal (465). Try to find a place where you can run on the grass or dirt, but if you *must* run on pavement, consider the temperature—if the sidewalk is hot, keep the dog off it.

**165. Dogs are a problem for me when I jog; they bark and chase after me. How can I safely take my own pet along?**  Keep your dog on a leash unless you're jogging in an area where you're reasonably sure there won't be a lot of other dogs or distractions.

**166. How can I protect myself and my dog from other dogs that try to pick fights**

*when I'm walking him?*   If you have trouble like this, I suggest you follow the lead of one of my clients—carry a cattle prod. It gives off a jolting electric sting, but it doesn't harm the animal (456).

*167.  Is it safe to ride a bicycle with my dog on a leash?*   This only works if you have a really good, obedient dog. If not, it can be trouble. The dog could be distracted by smells, other dogs, or people and pull away from you.

*168.  What are some alternatives to simply chaining my dog in the yard?*   A long leash hooked to a clothesline will give the dog a lot more room to run and explore. Another alternative is to use an outdoor cage about four feet wide and ten feet long. This kind of outdoor run, usually built with a concrete floor, gives the dog some exercise space but it still keeps the animal out of places in the yard that are off limits.

## Travel and Boarding

*169.  What can I do for a dog that gets motion sickness?*   You can expect some motion sickness from a puppy for the first few trips in a car (68). If you're going on a long trip and the dog is full-grown, you can give it motion sickness pills—an adult dose for dogs over forty pounds, and a child's dose for smaller dogs. If this doesn't help, your vet can prescribe a drug that will be more effective.

*170.  What precautions should I take when I'm going on a long car trip with my dog?*   The dog shouldn't eat for six hours before leaving. You *can* allow him water, though. While you're driving, stop every two hours and let the dog eliminate, exercise, and get some water. Feed the dog at night when you've stopped for the day. Be careful if your dog likes to stick his head out the window while the car is moving. This can be dangerous because he can get something in his eye, or he could even try to jump out. If the dog becomes restless while you're on a long trip, try increasing the exercise time at the next stop.

*171.  What can I do to calm my dog when we take her with us in the car? She jumps around and becomes very nervous during the ride.*   Try putting the dog in a collapsible cage. Dogs feel more secure in a kind of "den," and a cage can serve that purpose. If the dog is a very poor traveler and you must bring her with you, I would suggest you get some tranquilizers from your vet.

*172.  Is airplane travel safe for pets?*   Yes, provided certain precautions are taken. Small dogs and cats are usually allowed in the cabin, one for each class on commercial flights. The animals traveling in the baggage compartment are packed last. This area is pressurized, like the cabin, so that isn't a problem, although the temperature isn't controlled. However, this isn't a serious concern; I've never known a client's dog to suffer from the temperature at high altitudes. If the weather is particularly cold, the dog can be fitted with a sweater before the flight leaves. The big risk in the summer is that the dog will be left on a cargo loading area in the sun—airports can get very hot, and heat stroke is a real danger. The safest way to ship a dog in the summer is to send him on a night flight with no stops and no changes. Be sure to pick up the animal promptly; then give the dog a little water and let him rest.

**173. How should I prepare my dog for an airplane flight?**   Don't feed the dog for six hours before take-off. Give him water, but no food. If the dog is very excitable, I recommend that he be tranquilized; get the proper sedative from your vet.

**174. What health regulations can I expect to encounter when I'm traveling with my dog?**   You'll need a health certificate from a veterinarian before you can send your dog on most airlines. There are also a wide variety of requirements you may run into when you're crossing national borders. Mexico and Canada require any dog entering their territory to have had a rabies shot within the last year. Be sure to check on the regulations of any foreign country before you leave home.

**175. Are there regional disease problems I should be worried about when I'm traveling with my dog?**   If you're going to any coastal Atlantic area or to the central Mississippi River states, make sure your dog is on heartworm preventive medication (589). Start giving your pet regular doses of heartworm medicine a week before you leave, and keep it up for at least two months after your return. The medication will protect your dog from being infested by this dangerous parasite, but it works over a long period of time and it needs specific blood levels of medication in order to kill the parasite. Because of this, it's important that the dog be *kept* on heartworm pills for at least two months beyond the time of the animal's last possible exposure to the parasite.

**176. How well do dogs travel by boat?**   Most dogs don't have sea legs—they get sick. They may be all right if the weather is calm, but you still have to watch out for their dangerous habit of jumping *out* of boats. Once in the water, dogs don't always understand how to get back to the boat, and they may panic. Dogs *can* swim, but they aren't able to cover a lot of distance or swim for a long time, and some dogs (especially the toy breeds) have a real dislike for the water. All in all, boating with dogs usually isn't that good an idea. Certainly, though, this depends on the breed, the boat, and the type of water.

**177. Should I take my dog when I go backpacking?**   If you're going to an area where dogs are permitted, this is an excellent idea. However, there *are* some things to consider. Make sure the dog has a current rabies shot. And if your pet isn't used to the outdoors, you might take her on a leash to prevent any unpleasant encounters with skunks, porcupines, and badgers. The dog will also need supplies. In a dry area, you'll need to bring water and a bowl of some kind. Dry dog food is also a good idea because it's light. Some kind of flea protection will also be needed; a flea collar is probably the easiest. And you should search the dog for ticks after a day's exploring. One final reminder—be sure to keep track of your dog and not let her chase down wildlife. This kind of behavior has gotten dogs banned from a lot of natural areas.

**178. Do you recommend taking a dog on a camping trip?**   Yes. This can be a lot of fun. Just be sure to find out in advance whether the campground allows dogs inside. Also be sure to keep your dog on a leash while in the camping areas.

**179. I'm going to have to board my dog. What should I look for when I'm picking out a kennel?**   If the people who run the kennel want you to come back for a look later, be suspicious. You *must* see the place before you board your dog there. A good kennel operator should insist that every dog have a current distemper shot; if the kennel operator doesn't request this, he or she isn't really protecting your animal. The kennel should have an adequate concrete run where your dog can get some exercise—eight to ten feet is long enough. Also check for overcrowding, and give the place a sniff test—it should *smell* clean. Look the cages over to see that they're kept clean, and look at the condition of the animals that are housed there. For references, ask your vet, breeder, or groomer.

## The Older Dog

*180. How should we change our dog's diet as she gets older?*   Remember that different breeds age at varying rates, so a change like this should be calculated according to the dog's projected lifespan (244). Begin changing the dog's diet during the last quarter of the breed's average lifespan—about the age of 12 for most breeds, but 7 or 8 for the giant breeds. An elderly dog should be fed less overall bulk and receive higher-quality protein such as eggs, non-fat milk, and low-fat meat (poultry and fish). The aim in feeding your dog this kind of diet is to keep from overloading her kidneys (637). There are commercial dog foods made for pets with liver or kidney problems, but you can usually prepare a diet at home that's just as good (70). In general, you need only feed an older dog the minimal amount of protein required for a healthy diet. A vitamin and mineral supplement is also a good idea at this point in the dog's life. Rice or spaghetti can serve as bulk in the dog's homemade diet, but if you have a dog with a weight problem, you should probably substitute green beans, peas, or cottage cheese for spaghetti because they're lower in calories (70, 97).

*181. Should an older dog have veterinary check-ups more often?*   If the dog has any health problems, he should definitely be examined every six months. You should also discuss the problem with your veterinarian so that you'll know what danger signs to watch for. For instance, if the dog has heart disease and the cough that usually goes along with this ailment grows noticeably worse, that would be a sign that you should take the animal to your vet. If you wait, what *was* a treatable condition may cause irreversible harm.

*182. Our dog is old, and we worry about giving him too much exercise. Can this hurt him?*   Your aim should be to keep the dog active, but not let him overdo it. If he starts panting heavily, stop and let him rest. Remember, the dog is a bad judge of how much exercise is *too* much, and he'll push himself beyond his limit (158).

*183. Is it really true that you can't teach an old dog new tricks?*   It isn't easy. The dog develops patterns and habits over a long period of time, and changing her behavior when she's old can be very difficult. It isn't a good idea to even try unless it's absolutely necessary—you can confuse and worry an older dog by demanding a dramatic change of behavior late in life. Of course, there are times when the dog may forget an old lesson; for example, she may start barking a lot or defecating in the house. When this happens, you can use old training methods to re-establish what the dog already knew.

*184. Should we let our dog sleep inside now that he's getting older?*   Elderly dogs sleep a lot more than younger ones, and they need an environment that's protected from extreme temperatures (149). Try to find a place where the dog will be warm and dry, but won't be a lot of trouble for you. It doesn't have to be a place inside the house, as long as the animal is comfortable (150).

*185. We have an old dog that's begun to urinate in the house. Is this caused by senility?* Female dogs often have a hormonal problem that's marked by incontinence, a constant dribbling of urine. This is very different from just forgetting and urinating in the wrong place. That's why you should take the dog in for a physical check-up before you try to correct her behavior. If the problem is hormonal, it can be treated with estrogen supplements. Senility isn't usually a problem for a dog until about the age of 15. The only thing you can do is relocate the dog to a place where the animal won't hurt anything by urinating on the floor.

*186. As my dog has gotten older, his eyes have begun to cloud up. Are these cataracts?* Probably not. The appearance of a hazy, bluish cast to the eye (called nuclear sclerosis) is often a normal aging change for dogs. In most cases, the dog can dilate his eye to the point where he can see past this graying of the lens. Cataracts are an entirely different problem that's unrelated to age (632).

*187. Could old-age warts around a dog's face become a serious problem?*   Old dogs (especially poodles) often get a lot of wart-like skin tumors. They usually develop on the face, and less frequently on the dog's trunk. The growths pose no problem from a health standpoint, unless the dog is continually irritating them. If the dog happens to be undergoing surgery for some other problem, you may want to have the warts taken off at the same time, but otherwise they aren't worth the trouble and risk involved in putting an older animal under anesthesia.

*188. Our dog is getting old and has developed lumps on her skin that aren't the usual old-age warts—they're much larger. Can these be dangerous?*   There are a number of conditions that can cause a lump on a dog's skin. Cancer is one possibility (626), but it's more common for dogs to develop benign tumors and cysts as they grow old. The two main varieties are easy to tell apart, and generally they're quite harmless. *Sebaceous cysts* occur when a sebaceous gland in the dog's skin becomes plugged up and develops into a soft lump; these can be about as big as a quarter in size. No diet or special bath can prevent them, and the only real danger is that they may eventually become infected, open up, and then start draining. Sebaceous cysts can be removed surgically. You'll be able to recognize them by remembering that they're a part of the dog's skin—they move when the skin moves. *Fatty tumors*, on the other hand, occur under the skin—the skin can be pulled away from one of these blobs. Fatty tumors are just what the name implies, an enlarged pocket of fat. Like sebaceous cysts, fatty tumors are soft and pose no threat to the dog's health. They can be removed if they become too large, but otherwise it's better to leave them alone.

*189. Our dog is very old, and his breath smells terrible. What can we do to make it tolerable?*   This is usually caused by a build-up of plaque and bacteria on a dog's teeth, but in order to clean them he must be able to withstand anesthesia, something most elderly dogs (those over thirteen years old) lack the strength for. I always suggest that a dog have his teeth cleaned around the age of ten because most dogs are still in good health at that age, except for the larger breeds. If this isn't possible, you could try using a mouthwash gel or give the dog charcoal bones. You can relieve the situation somewhat by brushing the dog's teeth, but this is only effective if they've been professionally cleaned within the last year.

**190. What kinds of rheumatism and arthritis problems can we expect with an older dog?** Rheumatoid arthritis, or rheumatism, is a blood-related disease that has nothing to do with a dog's age (545), but osteoarthritis, the degenerative joint disease that comes with age, *can* be a problem. It's as prevalent in older dogs as it is in older people, although it isn't as severe because dogs don't notice the loss of paw dexterity and have twice as many legs to bear their weight. The first sign of trouble is usually a limp. Arthritis most often shows up in a dog's hips, less frequently in the knee or elbow, and occasionally in the carpus (wrist) and the tarsus (ankle). A dog with arthritic hips will hold his back legs close together with the feet pointing out and may be slow to rise or have trouble trying to sit or climb stairs. The problem grows worse with damp weather. It isn't curable, but the aches that come with arthritis *can* be treated. By and large, the best drug to use is aspirin, but it can't be given only when the animal seems to be in pain. To be effective, it has to be taken *daily* —one or two tablets for a twenty-pound dog once or twice a day, depending on the severity of the condition. Use a buffered aspirin to avoid upsetting the dog's stomach. A forty-pound dog may need the drug three or four times a day. Use the lowest dose possible at first, and always try to keep the amount as low as you can and still relieve the dog's suffering (308). For more severe problems, there are stronger drugs, such as corticosteroids, but they have some undesirable side effects, so you should try aspirin *first*, for about three months. Give it a chance to work before you switch to something stronger.

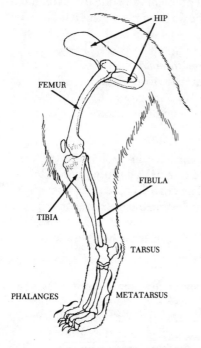

HIP

FEMUR

FIBULA

TIBIA

TARSUS

PHALANGES     METATARSUS

**191. Our dog is quite old, and we're thinking of getting a puppy. Will this cause a problem with the dog we have now?** This depends a lot on the disposition of the older dog. If he gets along well with other dogs, then there's probably no reason not to get a puppy. But if he isn't a very playful dog and has become cranky in his old age, a puppy could cause him some stress. Whatever the dog's temperament may be, an established dog in your home needs special consideration when a new puppy is introduced to the household, particularly if the dog is very old (25, 29). This kind of change has to be handled very carefully in order to keep the older dog from craving more attention and becoming confused by the situation.

**192. *At what point do you think an old dog's life should be ended to prevent unnecessary suffering?*** This is something for each individual to decide in consultation with the family veterinarian. My own feeling is that it's humane to take an animal out of suffering when the condition is painful and not likely to change (646). For instance, in cases of terminal cancer or the final, paralyzing stages of hip dysplasia, a dog's status may fluctuate within certain limits, but real improvement is impossible and pain is inevitable. One thing to remember is that a dog doesn't express chronic pain the way people do. A dog may cry out at a sudden, shooting pain, but she will endure a persistent ache without much display of emotion. That why the animal's *medical* condition is sometimes a better indication than her outward signs and actions of how much the dog may be suffering. A decision like this is a complex one that obviously involves more than health considerations. The relationship between the pet and her owner is a factor that shouldn't be ignored—it is in many ways a measure of the quality of the dog's life, and it deteriorates as the animal's condition worsens. When you sense that the link between you and your pet has broken down, the dog's suffering could be beyond the point of tolerance.

# PART II

# UNDERSTANDING YOUR DOG

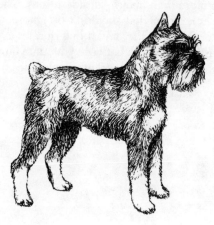

*Schnauzer*

## Dogs and Children
193-206

## The Problem Dog
207-240

## Dog Facts: Popular Beliefs, Common Behavior
241-255

## The Dog's Body and How It Works
256-279

# Dogs And Children

*193. What breeds of dog are good with children?* It depends an awful lot on the temperament of the individual dog, not to mention that of the child (22). Sex is also a factor because female dogs tend to be more docile than males. If I had to generalize, I'd recommend golden and Labrador retrievers. Good quality German shepherds are also well suited for children, as are springer spaniels, standard poodles, shelties, collies, German shorthaired pointers, terriers, and beagles, to name some of the better-known breeds. Generally speaking, it's better to stay away from toy breeds because they're often too small and high strung to fit in well with children. Other breeds with temperaments that may be too tense for the hectic demands of children are Irish setters, dalmatians, cocker spaniels, and miniature poodles. These breeds have a tendency to snap too easily when they're startled or excited. The giant breeds, even if their temperament is mild, can be intimidating to a child and hard to walk. The larger breeds also have a much shorter lifespan. St. Bernards are definitely *not* for children; under present breeding conditions, these dogs tend to have unpredictable personalities.

*194. People always say that pets are good for children. Beyond companionship, what can a dog contribute to a child's upbringing?* Having a dog is an excellent way to teach a child responsibility. Obviously, the child can also learn a great deal about respect for other living things by seeing, through close contact with a dog, that an animal has feelings too. Finally, a child's first encounter with death is likely to come about through the death of the family pet.

*195. How can I keep my child interested in our new dog?* Remember that the dog should be treated as a part of the family. Whenever possible, take the dog along on family trips and figure out some games you and the child can play that include the dog. In addition, children should be held responsible for some of the dog's regular care. Remember too that children often lose interest in a dog because of the poor example set by *adults*. If an adult doesn't want to take care of an animal, a child can't be expected to either.

*196. We adopted a grown dog from the animal shelter, and when we got him home he growled at the kids and ran from them. What should we do?* If a dog turns snappy and threatening around children this is an indication that it may have been mistreated by children in the past (20). There isn't much you can do except return the dog. Don't take a chance on having a child bitten. It may only be a minor injury, but it can result in a lifelong fear of dogs.

*197. Should I get a puppy to grow up with our new baby?* No. It's best for both the dog and the child to wait a little while. If the child is less than two years old, getting a puppy is a mistake—the dog is too young to know how to behave with a baby, and vice versa. A child who's about three years old usually has the maturity not to pull the dog's tail or mistreat the animal out of ignorance.

*198. We already have a dog and are expecting a baby. Can this be a problem?* To some extent it depends on the temperament of the dog—but most grown dogs will tolerate children, and most people know their dog well enough to be able to predict whether the animal can adjust to having a child in the house. The combination of a very young child and a grown dog is usually safe because the dog is mature enough to behave calmly around the child.

**199. How should we introduce the family dog to a new baby?** When the baby is born, the dog will naturally receive much less attention than she's used to. A couple of months before the baby is due, start tapering off the time you spend with her. This way there will be no sudden withdrawal of interest in the dog that could confuse her and generate resentment. Once the baby arrives, there's no reason why the dog can't be near the child while you're in attendance. Since dogs examine everything mostly by smell, encourage your pet to come up and sniff while you're holding the baby. This will create an association in the dog's mind between you and the baby. To preserve this link, never chase the dog away while you're holding the child. If the dog jumps up, you'll have to discipline her to break this habit (64).

**200. Is it all right for our toddler to play with the dog?** A young baby should never be left alone on the floor with a dog, simply because the child could get stepped on. Later, when the child begins crawling, there will still be a need for supervision because kids will often grab a dog in their efforts to stand up, and some animals may become frightened. If the dog doesn't like this kind of treatment from the child, separate them until the baby has gotten a little older.

**201. My children like to have the family dog sleep with them. Can this cause any medical problems?** There's no special risk, as long as the dog is clean and well cared for.

**202. How should a child approach a strange dog?** Teach children *never* to approach a stray dog. If a dog is with his master, the child should always ask if it's all right to pet the dog before going near him. Children should be taught not to approach a dog from the rear; dogs don't like to be surprised this way. It's also wise not to make sudden movements toward the dog. Instead, hold out your hand and let the dog come to you and sniff it.

**203. What kind of rules should we lay down for children concerning our dog?** Children should be taught not to make any sudden movements toward the dog—not to run at him, jump on him, or catch him off-guard while he's sleeping or eating. They should never tease a dog or pull any parts of his body. Although a dog should be trained to accommodate every member of the family (240), children should also be trained to treat the animal with respect.

**204. Isn't it a good educational experience for children to watch puppies being born?** It *can* be, but first there are some other important factors to consider. Breeding a dog requires a great deal of planning and involves added responsibility. Think about whether you'll be able to find good homes for the puppies, whether they'll be a burden to you and your family. If the litter proves to be a hassle, then this may be the *wrong* kind of educational experience for children, one that cheapens the birth process. As an alternative, contact local breeders to keep track of the gestation and birth of a litter.

**205. Aren't dogs carriers of a worm that can be very harmful to people, particularly children?** It is true that some dogs are infected with a parasite called roundworm that can be indirectly transmitted to human beings, but with some simple precautions the risk can be minimized. The worms are often transmitted to puppies during pregnancy or afterwards, so the first precaution should be to have your dog checked for worms yearly and treated when necessary (572). This treatment is nearly 100% effective. Even if the dog *does* have roundworms, people can't get them directly from the animal. Adult roundworms don't attack the human body; it's the *larval* form of the worm that's a problem—and the usual source of infestation for people is dog feces. This is why roundworms are more likely to be a problem in young children, who often go through a stage when they put everything in their mouths, including dirt. For this reason, small children shouldn't be allowed to play in an area where dog feces might be found (595).

**206. *Wasn't there some evidence found recently that connected distemper in dogs with multiple sclerosis in children?*** A study done in England first raised this question several years ago—there appeared to be some correlation between cases of distemper in small-breed dogs and multiple sclerosis in children living in the same homes. However, further investigation has turned up nothing to substantiate this.

## The Problem Dog

**207. *How can I stop my dog from chewing up the furniture while I'm away from home?*** If the dog is just chewing on one thing, you can use the same technique that's used for training puppies (62). But if you're coming home to a ransacked apartment, you've probably got a dog that's suffering from boredom. One way to ease this situation is to get a second animal to provide some companionship. Or you could embark on a training program. Start off by isolating the dog. Find an area where the dog can do little damage—a bathroom, laundry room, or garage—and put him in there while you're away. If you have a small apartment, get a big crate or cage, or a doghouse with a latching door (50, 51). When you have some time, on a weekend or a vacation, start working with the dog, testing his ability to leave things alone while you're out of the house. Let him out of his den, and leave for 10 or 15 minutes. When you come back, if you find something destroyed, put the dog back in his crate or pen. If everything is intact, praise him and pet him a lot. Next time, go away a little longer, and keep increasing your periods of absence by half an hour or so. Be sure to vary the time that you're away so the dog doesn't know when to expect you. When you can stay away for over four hours at a time with no resulting damage, you should be able to trust the dog by himself.

**208. *How can I prevent my dog from eating garbage?*** Eating garbage can be a very dangerous habit. Spoiled food and fat can cause severe stomach upset, as well as inflammation of the pancreas, a condition known as pancreatitis. There's also the chance that the dog will accidentally swallow poisons or will chew on bones. To prevent your dog from eating garbage, *never* allow her to roam, and make sure that she doesn't have access to your own garbage. If the dog eats garbage or feces (234) while you're walking her, get a piece of cheap meat and doctor it up with about half a bottle of hot pepper sauce. Be sure to hide the sauce so that the dog won't smell it. Stick the meat in a garbage can, and when the dog runs up, say, "No, don't eat!" She'll probably ignore you the first time, but it shouldn't take very long for her to learn to respect your opinion. You might also try using a cage- or cone-shaped muzzle on the dog when you walk her (145). Take her up to a piece of garbage she would ordinarily eat, and if she leaves it alone, praise her for her great self-control. Keep this up for a few days, and then walk her without the muzzle. Teach her that every time she eats while you're walking her, you'll make her wear the muzzle.

**209. Our dog obeys me, but ignores my husband. What can we do?** Your husband will have to establish his dominance over the dog. To do this, he should take over the routine duties that involve the dog so that the dog is *forced* to deal with him. You shouldn't even be present during this training. Before giving the dog his food, your husband should give him a few basic commands and withhold the food until the dog obeys. When the dog complies with the commands, reinforce this behavior with praise and petting, as well as with a bowl of food. If the dog is actually biting your husband, you'll have to get a muzzle (145). In the beginning, *you* should put the muzzle on the dog and then leave your husband and the dog alone. Your husband should then give the dog some basic commands, and when the dog listens and cooperates, the muzzle can come off. If there's any attempt to bite, the muzzle should go on again. Start with fifteen-minute sessions two or three times a day and increase them gradually to an hour. You should keep putting the muzzle on the dog for the first week; after that, it should be possible for your husband to do it. The crucial factor in all this is to be patient. You can expect this to take a *minimum* of a month.

**210. Is our dog likely to resent a new cat in the house?** Most dogs aren't bothered by the presence of a cat in their house. However, some dogs *do* chase cats. Ask a friend with a cat to bring her pet over for a visit so that you can see how your dog responds to it. This should help you decide whether you want a cat.

**211. My dog dashes out the door the minute it's opened. How can I break this habit?** Try baiting her a few times a day. Go to the door and open it a little. When she charges, don't slam the door, but close it suddenly, so that she's surprised. Do this two or three times a day for a week, and the dog should begin to think that she can never get through the door. If that isn't enough, get a long rope and tie it to the dog. Open the door and allow the dog to escape, then pull up abruptly after she's a few paces outside. Leave the rope on the dog's collar so you can step on it or grab it whenever anyone comes to the door, or when *you* want to go outside. The dog will never be sure if someone's at the end of the rope or not, and as she becomes less interested in dashing out the door you can gradually shorten the rope. After a few weeks, you can eliminate the rope entirely.

**212. My dog chases cars, joggers, bicyclists, pedestrians, anything that crosses our lawn. How can I stop this?** All you can do is pen the dog up, build a fence, or keep him on a leash or a chain. It's almost impossible to stop this kind of behavior because the dog is responding to his territorial instinct.

**213. Can a dog be trained to stay in a yard that's unfenced?** It's impossible. Dogs are territorial, but they don't recognize property lines and they love to roam, a practice that should be prohibited unless you live in a very rural area (216).

**214. My dog stays away from home for days at a time. How can I get him to stop wandering?** The dog can be restrained—penned, kept on a chain runner, or fenced—

and he can be castrated. In most cases, neutering does reduce the urge to roam, but if your dog is gone for days at a time he's probably been running with a pack—and neutering may not eliminate the problem. To stop this, you have to keep the dog at home and give him a little more attention than usual. Under no circumstances should he be allowed to run freely without close, continuous supervision.

*215. What advice do you have for someone who's trying to find a lost dog?* If the dog just wandered away, he probably hasn't gone very far. Put up a few posters in the neighborhood, offering a reasonable reward. Include a good picture of the dog, if you have one. Also check with the local animal shelter. Read the newspaper's lost and found column, and place an ad there. Another possibility is the city dog pound; stop by periodically to see what animals they've picked up. Good luck. (41)

*216. We live in the country, and our dog recently started chasing the farm animals. How can we control this?* Above all, don't let the dog run in a pack—this is where she often picks up these kinds of habits. Dogs in a pack will run down small wildlife as well as farm animals, and the more the dog runs with a pack, the more she will revert out of domestication. If the dog can't be controlled any other way, you'll have to keep her inside, in a pen, or tied up.

*217. When I'm leaving the house, our dog follows the car down the street. How can I train him not to do this?* Command the dog to "Stay!" and then drive away a few feet. If he doesn't follow, go back and praise him. Keep doing this until he gets the message. If this doesn't work, have an assistant tie a long rope to the dog's collar. The dog will chase after you, and the assistant should give the rope a hard pull when the dog gets to the end. Keep this up until the dog stops following the car.

*218. How can I stop my dog from digging in the yard?* Dogs love to dig, especially when the weather is hot. You'll just have to separate the dog from all that tempting dirt. The best way is to put the dog on a runner chain or fence the places that are off limits. If the dog is digging his way out of the yard, try putting bricks around the base of the fence. A second alternative is to try to condition the dog out of the digging behavior. Conceal yourself and wait for the dog to start digging. When the burrowing starts, make a loud noise with a can full of marbles or a starter's pistol. The dog should be startled. When the digging starts again, repeat the noise. The idea is to convince the dog that his digging is causing this loud, frightening sound. Be careful not to let the animal discover the source of the sound—you don't want to be associated with the noise because the dog will just wait until you're not around to do the dirty work. The dog has to decide that it's the *digging* that causes the sound.

*219. How do you train a dog to stop jumping the fence?* The best thing you can do is hire a professional trainer to temporarily electrify your fence. Unless you're an expert, don't try to electrify the fence yourself. The trainer can safely perform this service without the risk of giving the dog too much of a shock, and with no chance of accidentally shocking a person.

*220. My dog is thrown into a panic by the sound of firecrackers. Is there some way to control this?* This is often something you can plan for because fireworks are usually only used on holidays. Tranquilization is probably the most expedient solution. It's important, for safety's sake, only to use tranquilizers under the supervision of a vet. It also helps to keep the dog in a place that's as far as possible from the commotion, preferably in familiar surroundings.

*221. My dog is terrified of thunder and no amount of comforting seems to help when there's a storm. What can I do about this?* There's no way to plan ahead for a thunderstorm, so tranquilizing the dog is impractical. Anyway, by the time the drug took effect, the storm would probably be over. It's a better idea to train away the dog's fear. To do this, tape record a thunderstorm, or buy a sound-effects record of a violent storm. Play this at very low volume while you give the dog a lot of attention. Do this every day for about two weeks, increasing the length of time that the recorded thunder is playing, and gradually increasing the volume. This will teach the dog to associate good feelings with the sound of thunder, and take her fear away.

*222. We live on a very busy street. How can I stop my dog from being afraid of all the noise from the trucks and buses?* During a quiet time of the day, or during the evening, use the same technique that you'd use to calm a dog's fear of thunder (221).

*223. My dog barks all the time! How can I make him be quiet?* If the dog is just a puppy, you have a chance of disciplining this kind of behavior out of him (57). To correct this behavior in older dogs, you'll need a cone-shaped muzzle that's open at the nose (145). If the dog barks, put the muzzle on him, wait a few minutes until he's being quiet *by choice,* and then praise him. Take off the muzzle, and if he barks again, put it back on. If you keep this up, most dogs will learn not to bark.

*224. How can I teach my dog to be quiet while I'm not home? The neighbors say she barks all day.* Try the same technique that's used to train a dog not to dig in the yard—associate the barking with a noise that startles the animal (218).

*225. Isn't there a surgical method for silencing dogs? Do you recommend it?* Debarking is a painful procedure that's rarely done. In fact, it's been outlawed in some countries. It involves the removal of the dog's vocal folds (271), and it often proves to be a temporary remedy at best—the folds grow back and the dog begins barking again. I don't recommend debarking, even as a last resort. The owner of a noisy dog is better off simply finding another home for the animal. However, if you're determined to keep the dog, another possibility is an electric collar. This device delivers a jolt when the dog barks.

*226. Walking my dog is a daily struggle. How can I teach him to walk a straight line at a decent speed?* Some dogs are hard to leash train because of their natural, inbred inclination to range all around an area as they pass by. Other have just learned that they can bully their owner into doing whatever they want to do. The thing to remember is that dogs aren't like children; they won't ever "grow up" and suddenly act maturely. They have habits that you have to break—that's the only way to get behavior that's otherwise unnatural, but necessary if the two of you are going to get along. Nobody loves a domineering schnauzer.

For medium- and large-sized dogs, get a nylon choker. For small breeds, particularly Pomeranians and poodles (who suffer from a weak, easily collapsible trachea) use a harness. For dogs with especially thick necks, you might want to try a training

54

collar with blunt, hinged prongs designed to apply pressure without harming the dog (142). As you walk the dog, give him a little slack in the leash, and when he starts to strain and tug, take the leash and yank hard enough to knock the dog off balance. Gauge the strength of your yank to the size of the animal. Avoid starting a tug-of-war with the dog; this doesn't teach him anything, and it may even seem like a game. The point is to shock and surprise the animal, not hurt him. Yank without warning, and don't always do it at the same time. Couple this with positive reinforcement—lots of praise when the dog walks beside you.

**227. How can I keep my dog from running away when I let her off the leash to play? She won't come when I call her.** Get some rope and make a leash about twenty feet long. Let the dog run around until she gets out to the end of the leash, and then call her to you. If she doesn't come, slowly start pulling the dog in, still calling to her. Don't hurry, and maybe the dog will decide to come on her own. When the dog is at your side, praise her, pet her, and give her a treat. Do this five or six times, and the dog should get the idea that coming when you call can be rewarding. Let the dog off the leash to test her, and if she runs away again, catch her, tie her on the leash, and continue the exercise another five times. Eventually, the dog should learn to come when you call.

**228. How do you stop a male dog from trying to mount the wrong thing in the wrong place at the wrong time?** Push the dog down when he jumps up on you. Use your knee to emphasize the point; push forcefully, but not enough to hurt the dog. Give a sharp command—"No!"—followed by directions to sit and stay. Praise the animal when he complies. If you do this *every time* he attempts to mount, the dog should learn to behave himself. If the problem is chronic, mating can help, but this should never be the *only* reason for breeding a dog. Castration will also reduce this urge, particularly if it's done at an early age—from six to eighteen months (332).

**229. Our dog has been urinating on the living room furniture. How can we prevent this?** This is a male dog's method of staking out his territory. When you walk a dog, he won't urinate all at once; instead, he'll leave a little here and a little there. Urinating indoors is a natural variation of this behavior that's usually seen in small dogs that spend most of their time in apartments. If the dog is marking your sofa and chairs, there's no practical way to train it out of him because it isn't possible to catch him in the act and condition him to stop. It just isn't the same thing as housebreaking. Your options for correcting the situation depend on the age of the dog. Castration reduces the tendency in young dogs, and female hormones will act on older dogs. Of course, you can also try taking the dog outdoors more often.

**230. What can I do about a grown dog that suddenly loses her housebreaking?** Take note of how many times the dog has a bowel movement each day. If it's more than three times, there may be a medical problem, such as parasites or poor digestion. If medical problems are ruled out, this kind of behavior is usually caused by a change in the routine of the household. The dog becomes confused and a little anxious, and she starts forgetting her housebreaking. In this case, she'll need a few weeks of refresher training. Apply the housebreaking techniques you used when she was a puppy, confining the dog while you're away, and walking her regularly (59). It's rare for a dog to do something like this when her owner is at home, so it's probably safe to let the dog have the run of the house while you're there and only confine her when you're away. It may also help to change the dog's feeding schedule. If she's been eating in the morning and having a bowel movement in the afternoon when you're no longer home, start feeding her in the early evening so that you can walk her at night. A word of caution: Sometimes a person will rub the dog's nose in the mess on the floor to teach her not to defecate or urinate in the house. It doesn't work. There's no way the dog will figure out what the message is. She may act contrite, but only because your displeasure is obvious. There's no way the animal will connect the punishment with the crime. If you *do* catch the dog in the act, then you should command her to stop, make a loud noise by slapping a magazine beside her, or throw something at her like a shoe or a tin can with marbles in it—the idea is to startle but not hurt the dog. Then take her outside.

*231. My dog is so yappy and excitable that he's driving everybody crazy. He gets so overwrought that he can't control his bladder. How can I calm this animal down?* Try to train the dog to be more subdued. This will require consistency and some strictness on your part—the worst thing you can do with a dog like this is baby it. At feeding time, you should require the dog to sit quietly and be still before he's given his food. Do this exercise for five minutes at first, then increase the time to ten minutes, and then to fifteen minutes, which is probably about as much self-control as you can expect from a hyperactive dog, hungry or not. Reinforce the dog's calm behavior with petting and compliments, and ignore his manic outbursts. When the dog is running around, barking and carrying on, don't try to make him behave by talking to him in soothing, calm tones. He'll misunderstand your words and think of them as positive reinforcement for jumping around. He may even come to think that "hush" means "bark." Instead, give him firm, consistent commands to stop, and when he's quiet for a second don't immediately follow them up with petting and affection. You want him to *clearly* associate calmness with petting and affection. Whenever you catch him in a quiet mood, show him a lot of affection and tell him he's being a good, *quiet* dog. You may never completely cure the dog of his nervous habits, but the problem can usually be made manageable. If, however, you still have a lot of trouble with the dog, you should consult your vet about using a tranquilizer. Try the drugs *along with* further training.

*232. Is there some way to make the dog we got from the animal shelter relax and not be so afraid of strangers? He runs away and hides when new people come around.* This is called the "caged dog syndrome." It happens when a dog has spent two or three months without much human contact, often in a pen with other dogs that have dominated it. This creates some poor socialization habits, and it requires a lot of patience to eliminate them. The dog will usually become attached to at least one household member who should begin working to build up the dog's trust and confidence. Feed him, pet him, play with him, and after the dog begins to lose his fear, bring another person into the picture. This may take quite a while—from 6 to 24 months—but eventually the dog should be able to tolerate strangers without panicking. Even when this stage is reached, you shouldn't force a dog like this into a room full of strange people, nor keep him if you have small children around (196).

*233. We have a dog that behaves very submissively. When anyone approaches, she cowers, rolls over, and sometimes even urinates. The dog doesn't have any reason to be afraid. What can we do?*    This kind of behavior may be the result of nervousness or past abuse. To help stop it, make the dog greet you in a sitting position when you walk up to her. As you work with her, don't yell at her for cowering. Instead, make her sit up—and when she does, praise her. Always reward the desired, confident behavior with petting and praise, and show no response to the submissive actions. The dog *should* learn to relax.

**234. Sometimes I run my dog in a cow pasture, and he has the disgusting habit of taking bites out of cow patties. Why does he do this? How can I stop him?**    Dogs have a great ability to sort out different odors, but they don't usually play favorites with the things they smell. A lot of dogs will eat cow or cat feces because they're a source of high protein and fiber. However, this behavior can lead to stomach upset and can also expose the dog to internal parasites. To prevent this, use the methods for training a dog not to eat garbage (208).

**235. How can I stop my dog from eating his own feces?**    There's a product available in most pet stores that you can put in the dog's food—it makes his feces taste bad.

**236. My dog isn't normally aggressive, but he bites sometimes when he gets excited. How can this be controlled?**    This behavior is known as "fear biting." It's more common to certain breeds—the terriers, German shepherds, and toy breeds—and it's a difficult problem to manage. The dog isn't biting out of hostility or anger or because he has a bad temperament, but because he's learned to bite as a way of dealing with emotional stress. Usually such a dog will be docile with his owner, but not with other people. Unfortunately, the only solution to fear biting is to be prepared. Try to keep the dog out of the kind of situations in which he may bite; for instance, keep the dog away from children, who may play roughly with him. Instruct people about the dog's habits and the kinds of things that bother him. Working with fear biters takes a lot of patience. You have to go slowly with them and build their trust when you're trying to do things that make them nervous, such as giving them a shot or clipping their nails. If you have small children and your dog is a fear biter, the best solution is probably to adopt the dog out to another household.

**237. Why does my Doberman pinscher keep gnawing and drooling on his side?**    Your dog is probably afflicted by a harmless but bizarre trait that's found in Doberman pinschers. They don't bite or cause any irritation; they just make the fur very wet and puzzle a lot of owners. It's a kind of nervous habit that can be reduced with a sedative. Although this helps, the habit is likely to recur. And although it's not pleasant, it's really nothing to worry about.

**238. What can be done about a hostile, biting dog?**    Some dogs have been almost *encouraged* to be attack dogs—they haven't been taught the professional ethics of a good guard dog. Instead, they've grown up to dislike strangers, bark a lot, and bite when they get the chance. After the first couple of incidents, it should be obvious to the owner that such a dog is not under control. There are only two options—seek a professional trainer or adopt the dog out to a more appropriate setting.

**239. What can I do to stop a big dog from gobbling up his food too fast?**    The best thing to do is divide the dog's daily meal into thirds, and give the dog three meals a day, or a portion every half hour, whichever is more convenient. Eating too fast can be a dangerous habit for a large dog (88).

**240. How can I keep a dog from growling at me when I pick up his food bowl?** As part of the dog's basic training, everybody in the household should come and take food or a toy away from the puppy so that he gets used to the idea that people can take his possessions away at any time. If the dog is grown and behaves very aggressively when you reach for his food bowl, you *must* confront the dog and stop this behavior. In an extreme case, you may even have to wear protective gloves. Be calm and firm with the dog, and show him that growling and biting over food or toys will not be tolerated. Remember that children should *never* try to take anything away from a strange dog. This could easily result in a bad bite.

## Dog Facts: Popular Beliefs, Common Behavior

**241. What's the smartest breed of dog?** That depends on your definition of intelligence. I.Q. tests have indicated that miniature poodles are the smartest breed, but the results of tests like these are questionable because they may stress certain qualities and ignore others. For instance, miniature poodles are very quick to gauge people's moods and emotions, and they learn training routines quickly. However, miniature poodles tend to be nervous dogs, unable to adapt well to sudden changes. Other breeds that are more difficult to train— but less sensitive to your moods— may be able to adjust much more easily to changes around them. So an evaluation of a dog's mental capabilities depends on what you value in a dog.

**242. Which animal is smarter, a cat or a dog?** At the risk of being accused of ducking the question, the truth is that this is like asking which tastes better, cheese or apricots. Dogs and cats occupy different ecological niches, and it's not easy to make any valid comparisons between them.

**243. Is it true that one year in a dog's life is the equivalent of seven human years?** It isn't that simple. The aging rate of dogs varies from breed to breed (244), and it changes with the stages of the dog's life. A puppy matures very quickly compared to a human. In the young adult and middle years, a dog's aging process slows down to one year for about four or five human years, a rate that remains fairly consistent for the remainder of the dog's life.

|  | AGE EQUIVALENTS |  |  |
| --- | --- | --- | --- |
| *DOG* | *HUMAN* | *DOG* | *HUMAN* |
| 8 months | = 13 years | 7 years | = 44 years |
| 1 year | = 16 years | 9 years | = 52 years |
| 2 years | = 24 years | 11 years | = 60 years |
| 3 years | = 28 years | 13 years | = 68 years |
| 5 years | = 36 years | 15 years | = 76 years |

**244. Do the lifespans of different breeds vary?** Yes, they do. The dogs with the shortest lifespans are the biggest ones, the giant breeds like Great Danes, Newfoundlands, and St. Bernards. Any dog over 200 pounds ages quickly—they're old at age six and live an average of about nine years. On the other hand, the type of dog with the longest lifespan is the typical, mid-sized mutt. These hardy genetic mixtures easily live to be fourteen or fifteen years old, and sometimes much older.

**245. What breed is the worst when it comes to fighting with other dogs?**  Chows are the most aggressive of the fighting dogs; bull terriers, huskies, and malamutes also share this trait. The males of these breeds tend to be extremely aggressive toward other males—behavior that's an outgrowth of pack life and the need to dominate. If they're allowed to roam, these dogs will often get into fights with other dogs, and it isn't uncommon for them to kill smaller dogs with little or no provocation. This combative trait manifests itself at an early age, and the most effective way to reduce it is to have the dog neutered. It's also important to have the dog completely leash trained.

**246. What was the worst dog fight you've ever heard of?**  It happened when two roaming German shepherds jumped a backyard fence and ganged up on an Irish wolfhound. The owner of the wolfhound found his dog near death, with one German shepherd already dead and the other severely crippled. He rushed the wolfhound to my office, and the animal died not long after he arrived. The wolfhound's body was ripped and bleeding; there were about 150 puncture wounds. It was a bloody lesson in the danger of letting dogs roam at will.

**247. I've heard that Doberman pinschers are extremely unpredictable and have a history of unprovoked attacks, even against their owners. Is this true?**  No. This story got started not because of a problem with the dog but because of a failure on the part of some Doberman owners. Dobermans have a well-earned reputation as guard animals, but some people have used them for this purpose without giving them proper training. There will always be some dogs in any breed that have temperament problems, and Dobermans may have been overbred at one time—and this created a situation in which some unsuitable dogs were used as guard animals. Responding to this problem, breeders have done an excellent job in recent years of selecting mates for even temperament, and as a result the Doberman breed has become a more consistently docile dog.

**248. Why do dogs bury bones?**  In the wild, dogs range over a lot of territory. They bury things so they can come back and get them later.

**249. When my dog gets ready to lie down she turns a couple of circles first. Why does she do this?**  Your dog is instinctively making a nest. In the wild, dogs lived in tall grass, so at night they would turn and press the grass down to make a place to sleep.

**250. Is it true that a dog won't urinate where he sleeps?**  It depends on how the dog is cared for, particularly in the case of a puppy. If a dog is confined in a small area, both the pen and the dog must be kept clean. Otherwise, the dog's habit of not fouling his nest can be eliminated by the constant smell of urine. For instance, if a puppy urinates in a cage, then steps in it, gets it on his fur, and becomes accustomed to the smell, he'll stop noticing the smell. He has to notice a *difference* in smell between his sleeping place and the spot where he urinates in order to maintain this sanitary behavior.

*251. Why do dogs smell each other's rear ends when they meet?* Dogs don't recognize each other so much by structure and color as by smell. They sniff each other's rear because the anal scent glands are located there, serving as a kind of biological name-tag for each dog.

*252. How much do dogs communicate with each other by barking?* Very little of dog communication is oral. They use body language, eye contact, and gestures to get across feelings and moods to each other. The growl is a vocal threat used among dogs, but its accompanying facial expressions, postures, and movements can change its meaning entirely. A threatening dog will approach another dog and communicate hostility by eye-to-eye contact; approaching head-on, he'll move straight at the other dog, growling and snarling, with his ears forward. If all these signals are present but the ears are back, the dog is signifying a less hostile warning. In response to these threats, a submissive dog will roll over on his back, avoid eye contact, and allow the dominant dog to stand over him. The dog may also urinate or whine. If two dogs are friends, they'll greet each other, sniffing rear ends, and then possibly alternate urinating on some nearby object, sniffing this marking. They won't face each other head on; instead, they'll stand off to the side of each other. They may bark, but not threateningly.

*253. Why do dogs eat grass?* Nobody knows but the dogs. It's hard to say if they eat grass to make themselves throw up, or if they throw up because they eat grass. And dogs eat grass even if they aren't sick; they seem to like the consistency of it. Whatever the reason for this behavior, eating grass isn't good for dogs. The grass itself is usually harmless, but often the blades are loaded with parasite ova.

*254. Is it true that people who own dogs have fewer heart attacks?* A recent study showed that coronary patients who owned dogs lived longer after their heart attacks than people who had no pets. This increased lifespan was attributed to the possibility that having a dog as a companion eased the patient's tension. This doesn't mean that it's a good idea to go out and get a puppy if you just had a heart attack—after all, raising a puppy can be a strain. But if you have a dog already, it may be nice to know that your pet can be a help.

*255. Are dogs now being trained to help deaf people in much the same way that seeing-eye dogs help the blind?* Yes. Hearing-ear dogs are now being placed with deaf people. The animals are trained to serve as the individual's link to sounds—to tell their masters when someone is at the door, when the alarm clock goes off in the morning, when the telephone is ringing, and so on.

## The Dog's Body and How It Works

*256. Are there physical signs that can be used to estimate a dog's age?* Dogs aren't like horses; you can't accurately gauge their age by changes in their teeth. However, there *are* some reliable but less precise clues to a dog's age than can be seen in its teeth—signs of wear, discoloration, and tartar accumulation. Pups acquire all their baby teeth when they're between four and eight weeks old. These teeth are thin and extremely sharp. By the time the young dog is six months old, it will have lost these teeth and replaced them with thicker, broader permanent ones. From this point on, it becomes more difficult to figure the dog's age by its teeth because the condition of the teeth depends a lot on the dog's diet, and because different breeds have different rates of aging. However, it's usually a safe bet that the dog is less than a year old if the teeth are still sharp and as white as a smile in a toothpaste commercial. From the ages of one to three, you can expect to see a mild tartar build-up on the dog's canine teeth (fangs) around the gums, a loss of the sharp points, and the first signs of dulling on all the teeth. From the ages of three to five, the tartar accumulation will become apparent on all the teeth, and the back molars will begin to yellow. During the fifth, sixth, and seventh years, the teeth will show a thickening of the tar-

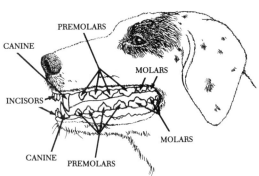

tar stain and a slight recession of the gums. The flat, front teeth (incisors) will also wear until they lose their straight edge and become more oblong, worn on the inside and buckled outward. From seven to ten years of age, there will be a heavy tartar build-up and a marked gum recession. Dogs over ten years old will also usually have a gray muzzle, missing teeth, and a bluish cast to their eyes from changes in the lenses (186).

**257. How many teeth does a dog have?** A dog has 28 baby teeth and 42 permanent adult teeth. Dogs begin to lose their baby teeth when they're about three months old, and they have a full set of adult teeth by the age of six months—the age at which a dog in the wild begins to fend for himself and fight for rank within the pack.

**258. What's the dog's strongest sense?** Dogs have two very accurate, finely tuned senses—smell and hearing. A good tracking hound can stay on scents so faint that they're the equivalent of a drop of vinegar in a thousand gallons of water. A dog's sense of hearing is capable of picking up noises long before they're audible to a human, and a dog can also hear sounds in pitches outside our range. All this sometimes makes the animal seem to have a kind of extrasensory perception when in fact he's just listening very closely for a particular sound. By the way, dogs with ears that stand up have the greatest hearing ability, better than breeds with long, floppy ears. The pointed ears are natural cups for bringing in the sound, and the tiny muscles that control them allow the dog to move his ears in several directions.

**259. Why have some dogs developed long, floppy ears?** This kind of ear is found mostly in hunting breeds. It may have evolved as protection in the brush to keep burrs, thorns, and other damaging objects out of the dog's ears during the chase.

**260. Are there any smells that dogs find offensive?** Yes. They don't evaluate things for freshness or rottenness, but they do avoid very bitter or caustic smells, such as ammonia and other chemicals. They also keep away from smoke.

**261. Is it true that dogs sweat only from their tongues?** No. That's saliva that's dripping off a dog's tongue when she's panting. Dogs drool so much because they have to keep their mouths open and breathe to expire internal body heat. The only place dogs sweat is on their noses and the pads of their feet. This is why they have so little tolerance for heat (460).

*262. Isn't a dog's mouth a lot cleaner than a person's mouth?* The canine mouth is populated by the same hordes of bacteria we have in our own mouths. Making matters worse is the fact that dogs have no regular dental hygiene and eat all kinds of questionable substances. Dogs, like presidential candidates, should never be kissed on the lips. You never know what those lips were doing before they smiled at you.

*263. Do whiskers serve any important function on a dog's face?* The whiskers on a dog's face are probably vestiges from an earlier stage of evolution. A dog's whiskers are just specialized hair.

*264. How good is a dog's sense of sight?* Much poorer than a human's. Dogs can't distinguish objects in detail at a distance of more than about a hundred feet. A dog lives mainly in a world of scent, exploring and reacting to smells much more than he does to sights. This is one reason why dogs sometimes respond strangely to people, places, or objects that may seem to be quite harmless and ordinary to us. They may be reacting to the smell of another dog, or to scents that remind them of past negative experiences. A dog's visual limitation can also cause the animal to misinterpret a person's actions. The dog may not be able to distinguish between a threatening gesture and an unrelated movement, and may simply respond to *any* activity. In the case of a bad-tempered dog, this can cause an unprovoked attack.

*265. Are dogs color blind?* It appears that dogs see color in the same kind of limited way as color-blind humans—making out shades and seeing some differences in tones and colors, but not with the sharpness and variety of normal human vision.

*266. What's the function of that movable covering under the dog's eyelid?* The third

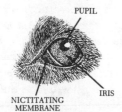

PUPIL

IRIS

NICTITATING
MEMBRANE

eyelid, or nictitating membrane, is there for added protection of the eye. Most of the time, it's visible in the inside corner of the dog's eye, and it moves up automatically when the eye is exposed to a chronic irritation, such as excessively bright light, wind, or debris. The dog can't blink this membrane the way he can his other eyelids—the nictitating membrane functions by reflex action (283).

*267. Can I tell if a dog has had a litter by looking at her?* A dog with slightly enlarged breasts probably has had a litter. If she has small, rather undeveloped breasts and her vulva is also small and a little bit retracted, there's a good chance that the dog was spayed before she was a year old.

*268. Is there any medical significance if a dog has an odd number of nipples?* None whatsoever. The normal number is ten, but sometimes a dog will be born with eleven, and less frequently with nine.

*269. Do male dogs have nipples?* It's surprising the number of times I've been asked this question. People never consider the simple fact that the male dog has breasts just like the female, and would produce milk just like a pregnant bitch if he were given the proper mixture of female hormones.

**270. Is it true that some dogs are born with both male and female sex organs?**   This does occur sometimes, mostly with schnauzers. The dog won't have two different sets of external genitalia, but there *can* be one or more reproductive glands of both sexes. When the animal has two complete sets, it's referred to as an hermaphrodite; with one and a half sets of organs, it's called a pseudohermaphrodite.

**271. What kind of vocal ability does a dog have?**   Dogs don't have vocal cords like those that people use when they talk. Instead, dogs have more rudimentary organs known as vocal folds, which make a very limited range of sounds.

**272. What breeds run fastest?**   Greyhounds, whippets, and salukis. These dogs can reach speeds of 45 miles an hour.

**273. What's the tallest breed of dog?**   The Irish wolfhound stands about 36 inches at the shoulders and stretches around seven feet from head to foot when standing up on two feet. Full grown, these dogs weigh about 175 ponds.

**274. What breed of dog is the smallest?**   At a pound and a half, the teacup Yorkshire terrier is the least amount of dog that money can buy.

**275. Were small dogs originally bred for any special purpose?**   Yes. The small terrier breeds were first developed to hunt for rats and small game. They have the obvious advantage of being able to get down into holes, to flush out the quarry or to rid the farmer's barn of rats. The dachshund, with its long body, short legs, and pointed snout, was adapted especially to hunt burrowing game.

**276. What breeds are biggest, and how big do they get?**   Great Danes, bull mastiffs, and St. Bernards are the heavyweights of the canine world, with St. Bernards weighing in as high as 275 pounds.

**277. How hard can a big dog bite?**   A really large dog, one of the giant breeds, can exert as much as 500 pounds of jaw pressure. That's more than enough to crush a man's arm, and if the dog is really angry this power can be combined with a tearing action that can leave the animal's victim in shreds.

**278. Do dogs have different blood types?**   Yes, they do, but they aren't as complex as ours are. Usually, if an emergency transfusion is required the blood type is nothing to worry about. The health risks of mixing types are very minor. There are two basic dog blood types: A-positive and A-negative, with some other factors that further subdivide them medically. A-negative is the universal type, the blood that can be transfused into any dog with no difficulty whatsoever. Animal hospitals usually keep a dog with this type of blood on hand as a donor dog for transfusions. The dog may have been abandoned by his owner, or he may have been a stray. He's tested regularly to make sure he's free of diseases.

**279. Could a dog's blood be used in a human transfusion?**   No. Different species can't swap blood. This would be fatal.

# PART III

# GENERAL MEDICAL CARE

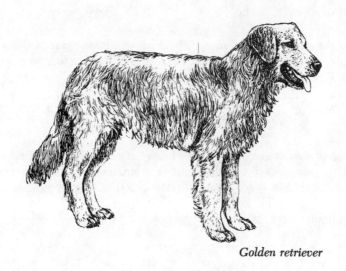

*Golden retriever*

Preventive Medicine: Monitoring Your Dog's Health
280-293

Home Medical Care
294-318

Spaying and Castration
319-334

# Preventive Medicine: Monitoring Your Dog's Health

**280. *How often should my dog have a veterinary check-up and what should it include?*** A yearly examination is usually enough, unless the dog is very old or suffers from some chronic, serious problem. Each annual visit should include a DHLP vaccination (281). Rabies shots can be given yearly or as infrequently as once every three years, depending on the type of vaccine that's used. During the yearly exam, the vet should also check your dog's teeth for tartar build-up, examine the animal's ears for wax accumulation and signs of infection, listen to the chest for heart problems and lung abnormalities, check the abdomen and a female's breasts for tumors, clip the dog's nails if they need trimming, and check the anal scent glands for signs of trouble. These operations—along with other indications, such as the dog's appearance—should allow your vet to make a general assessment of your pet's health.

**281. *What protection does my dog get from one of those annual four-in-one vaccinations?*** This is an excellent preventive medicine that combines distemper vaccine with protection from hepatitis, leptospirosis, and parainfluenza (kennel cough).

**282. *How can you tell if a dog is in pain?*** Acute pain is obvious. If a dog has a sprained joint and you touch it, the animal cries out. But chronic pain is expressed more subtly. For example, the dog's disposition may change. A normally mild dog may become ill-tempered, or a mean dog may turn lethargic. A dog that's in pain may be less willing to move around or walk up steps, and will generally seem less active. The animal may take on a depressed look and have a reduced appetite.

**283. *What can you tell about a dog's physical condition by looking at his eyes?*** Of course, eye diseases are the most obvious, but other diseases also affect this part of the body. Some dogs suffer from constantly draining tears, and this may be a normal condition (501), but for other dogs it can be a sign of an upper respiratory or sinus infection. A blue cloudiness of the eyes is an early sign of hepatitis, and one indication of anemia is a paleness of the normally pink conjunctiva, the membrane surrounding the eye. If the dog is dehydrated, his eyes may take on a sunken and dull look, and the third eyelid won't completely retract (266). In general, if a dog is feeling run-down his eyes will lose some of their gloss.

**284. *Is it true that the condition of a dog's coat reflects his general health?*** There's some truth to this. Hair regenerates quickly, and it requires protein as it grows, so a poor-quality coat can indicate malnutrition, metabolic deficiencies, parasites, or other internal disorders. If your dog's coat stops being shiny and becomes dull, sparse, or flaky, this is a sign that something could be wrong.

**285. *Can you tell anything about a dog's health from his nose?*** No. You can't judge a dog by his nose, although it may reflect some symptoms. For instance, when the dog has the flu a mucus discharge will be present—but even this will be only *one* danger sign among several. The proverbial cold, wet nose of a healthy dog can be normal, or it may be the result of a respiratory problem. Or the dog's nose may be wet just because this is one of the two places a dog sweats (the other is his paw pads). By the same token, a dog's nose isn't a good indicator of a high temperature. A more accurate place to check for fever is the stomach.

*286. Does the color of a dog's feces tell you anything about the animal's health?*
Sometimes it provides a clue. Of course, if the dog has been eating processed dog food or colored biscuits, there may be dyes in them that can tint the animal's stool. However, there are some natural indications to look for. A *pale, chalky* stool is a sign that there may be a pancreas problem. *Dark, tarry* feces is a sign that blood is coming from the small intestines, and this could mean the dog has worms or a number of other problems, including cancer. *Mucus* in a dog's stool is a sign of an inflamed colon, either from whipworms or from an irritation to the colon, perhaps from poorly digested food. Another sign to look for is *blotches of blood* in the feces. The blood will be clearly identifiable. Blotches of blood usually originate in the large intestine and they could be caused by a minor irritation such as a bone or rough food. In these cases the problem should clear up within 24 hours. If not, have the dog checked by your vet. Actually, the solidity of the feces is a more significant indication of the dog's health than the color. They should be somewhat firm, and not runny or diarrheic (496).

*287. How often will a normal dog urinate every day?*   Three to six times a day is average for females. A male will save up urine and use it to mark territory, excreting small amounts throughout his range. Because of this, there's no specific, normal amount or frequency of urination for a male dog.

*288. What's the normal body temperature for a dog?*   A dog's normal body temperature is 101 to 102°F. (38.3 to 38.8°C.). If the dog is very excited while you're taking his temperature, the reading could be as high as 102.5°F. (39.2°C.). (297)

*289. What's the highest body temperature a dog can tolerate?*   A body temperature of 104°F. (40°C.) is very high for a dog, and it could indicate a serious infection, either internal or external. If the dog is suffering from heat stroke, his internal temperature may reach 106°F. (41.1°C.), and if it remains there for thirty minutes or more, the dog will either die or suffer serious brain damage (462).

*290. What's a normal pulse rate for a dog?*   At rest, the dog's pulse should be about 120 beats a minute (298). However, this can vary greatly, and the pulse can easily go up to 200 beats a minute if the dog gets excited. Such a high rate isn't evidence by itself that there's any health problem. If your dog seems to have a high resting heart rate, other signs must be considered before deciding there's something wrong.

*291. What does it mean if my dog has an abnormal heart rate?*   A fast, weak heart rate can be a sign of anemia—the circulatory system lacks enough red blood cells to carry oxygen to the dog's tissues, so the heart compensates by pumping faster. A fast, weak heartbeat may also indicate internal bleeding or heart failure—the heart may be trying to compensate for a loss of blood pressure. If you suspect this may be the case, check the dog's gums to see if they're pale; that's another indication of internal bleeding. Drug reactions, overexcitement, and a number of different heart diseases also cause an abnormally fast heartbeat. Other possible causes include a faulty heart valve or a tumor that may be causing hyperthyroidism.
    In the case of a significant abnormality in the dog's heart rate, try the following test. Take the dog's pulse (298) and feel his heartbeat at the same time. If the heart is pumping rapidly but the pulse is slow there's some malfunction that's keeping the

blood from getting through the heart chambers and into the arteries. This condition will usually be accompanied by lethargy, and it's *dangerous*. The animal should have a professional examination quickly.

**292. Do dogs undergo the same kinds of stress that cause high blood pressure in people?**   Yes. I'm sure this is true, especially for city dogs. Of course, we can't monitor the blood pressure of dogs very easily, so we don't really know much about the effects of stress on their cardiovascular systems. Dogs don't suffer from heart attacks, but it does seem obvious to me that city dogs must experience mental and physical stress from being confined for large amounts of time. Remember too that dogs are very territorial, and whenever a dog goes for a walk in the city he encounters territorial smells left by dozens of other dogs, so this must also bother him.

**293. How can you tell if a dog is becoming dehydrated?**   A slight dryness of the gums and mouth is an obvious sign. Another test is to pick up the skin on the dog's back. If it snaps back into place right away, the animal is all right. If the skin stays up and goes back down very slowly, the dog is becoming dehydrated. The dog's eyes are another indicator of dehydration (283).

## Home Medical Care

**294. What kind of records should I keep if my dog is sick?**   Make note of any symptoms, such as seizures, vomiting, and so forth, and any medication you give the dog. Be as accurate and specific as possible. You'll be a great help to your veterinarian if you note the animal's symptoms in detail. For example, if the dog is vomiting, try to record how many times the vomiting has occurred and how long it's been going on. What was produced? Was it regurgitated food or blood or bile? These kinds of observations can be very helpful.

**295. What kind of medical supplies will I need to keep on hand for my dog?**   You shouldn't have to buy anything that a well-equipped medicine cabinet doesn't have already. Here's a check-list: cotton, gauze (four-inch by four-inch pads), adhesive tape, antiseptic solution or peroxide, boric acid eyewash, tweezers or hemostats (surgical clamps), scissors, alcohol, stomach antacid, cough medicine, aspirin, a rectal thermometer, an eyedropper, antibiotic ointment or powder, mineral oil, petroleum jelly, an emergency poison antidote kit, and possibly a snakebite kit.

**296. What kind of antiseptic solution should I use on my dog?**   Just about any mild antiseptic is fine, including those available at the drugstore for human use. Alcohol is too strong and stinging; it will make the dog unnecessarily hard to handle. Hydrogen peroxide is good for a sore that's dirty and needs to be washed out and opened, but continued use after this first cleansing will interfere with healing. Antibiotic ointments and powders are also good for many external cuts and sores; the powders are particularly good for moist wounds and skin irritations because they have a drying effect and the dog is less likely to lick them off.

**297. How do you take a dog's temperature?**   Lubricate a rectal thermometer with petroleum jelly and insert a third to a half of it into the dog's rectum. Hold it in for at least a minute in order to insure an accurate reading. Unless the dog is very small, this operation will probably require two people, one to take the temperature, and one to hold the dog and try to keep him calm.

**298. How do you take a dog's pulse?** The best spot for taking a dog's pulse is his femoral artery, located on the inside of the thigh of one of his back legs, up high next to his body. You should be able to feel the large leg bone called the femur; the femoral artery will be just in front of it. Press your finger over the femoral artery. Another place where you can find a pulse quickly for a dog in shock is the bottom of the dog's tongue (303).

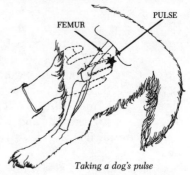

*Taking a dog's pulse*

**299. How do you take a dog's blood pressure?** The only way to take a dog's blood pressure is to stick a catheter into one of the animal's arteries, so obviously it isn't a routine procedure for veterinarians. There just doesn't seem to be a way to fit a measuring device on the body of a dog, keeping in mind the fact that dog's bodies can range so greatly in size.

**300. What's the best way to take a urine sample?** For males, use a wide-mouthed jar. While you're walking the dog, reach down quietly and collect about a quarter of a cup of urine. For female dogs, just place a flat pan under the animal when you're walking her. Be sure to move calmly and quietly so you don't startle her.

**301. How should I collect a stool sample?** Just scoop it up and place it in a jar or a plastic bag. (You won't need more than about a tablespoonful.) Refrigerate the sample if you're not going to take it to the veterinarian's office on the day it's collected.

**302. How can I weigh my dog? He won't fit on the bathroom scales.** Weigh yourself, then pick up the dog and weigh again. Subtract the lower weight from the higher one, and the remainder is the weight of the dog.

**303. How do I give my dog a pill?** If the medicine is in a capsule, it helps to wet it first. This makes the capsule slippery and easy to swallow. However, just the *opposite* is true for pills. Wetting them first only makes them begin to dissolve, and then the dog tastes them and usually puts up a fight. To give your dog a pill *or* a capsule, hold her muzzle with one hand and tilt her nose up a bit. Stick your thumb in the

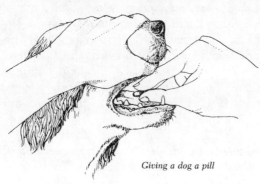

*Giving a dog a pill*

space between her canine tooth and her first molar and press it against the roof of her mouth—this will force her to keep her mouth open. With your other hand, drop the medication as far back in the dog's mouth as you can, making sure that it's *on top* of her tongue, not under it. Then hold her mouth closed and gently massage her throat until you feel her swallow. If your dog likes peanut butter (or lunch meat or cheese or whatever) you can often trick her into swallowing a pill along with her favorite snack.

**304. What's the easiest way to get a dose of liquid medicine into my dog?** An eyedropper or an old syringe with the needle removed is the best bet. You could also use a tablespoon if neither of these is available, although the spoon is harder to work with. If you can get an eyedropper that has liquid measures on it, this would be the best. For larger amounts, you can use a turkey baster. If a baster is all you have, you can usually dilute smaller amounts of medicine with water so that the solution will

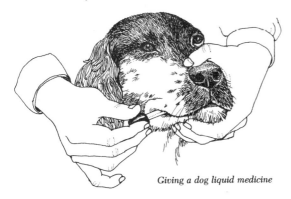

*Giving a dog liquid medicine*

draw into the baster. (Be sure, though, to check with your vet before you dilute any medicine because in some cases this can destroy its effectiveness.) *Never* use anything made of glass to administer medicine; this can be very dangerous. Once you've gotten the medicine ready, hold your dog's snout in your free hand. Dogs have a gap just behind their canine teeth—you can poke the medicine through this gap while you're holding the dog's mouth shut. Keep his mouth shut until he swallows. The animal may struggle if the medicine doesn't taste very good, but usually this method gets enough in him to do the job. When you're giving the dog prescription drugs, don't try to compensate for any medicine you may have spilled by exceeding the dose. However, if you're giving the dog a common remedy, such as an antacid, and most of it goes out the side of his mouth, just reload and give him some more. It helps to do this in the kitchen or bathroom—cleaning up will be easier.

**305. Can't you just put most medicines in the dog's food and let him take them that way?** Ask your vet first—some antibiotics are deactivated by certain foods. Remember too that the dog may be so sick that he doesn't have an appetite, or he may be finicky about what he eats—he may pick around the medicine or skip eating completely, losing out on nutrition *and* medication at the same time.

**306. What's the best way to apply medicine to a dog's eye?** You may need help to keep the dog's head still if your pet is the nervous type. For eye drops, hold the bottle above the eye and press gently above the upper lid with your free hand. This will retract the lid. Squeeze in the drops, taking care that they actually *drop* into the eye—the bottle mustn't touch the eye; otherwise, the medicine can become contaminated. If you're applying powder or ointment, press just below the eye to turn down the lower lid. Then apply the medication on the inside of the lid.

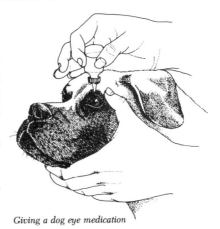

*Giving a dog eye medication*

*307. Are human antibiotics effective when they're given to dogs?*   Yes. In fact, there are very few antibiotic drugs that are made specifically for animal use. About 80 percent of the drugs we use on dogs are identical to their human counterparts.

*308. What other human medications can be given safely to dogs?*   Stomach antacids can be used for treating diarrhea and vomiting (495). Laxatives and mineral oil are acceptable for treating constipation, as are glycerine suppositories. Of course, if the dog is showing signs of stomach pain, is vomiting excessively, or is lethargic, you should take him to your vet—the problem could be something more serious than constipation (500). Cold capsules can be given to a dog (518), and liquid cough medicine is also useful, but be careful of the ones that contain sedatives (codeine and phenobarbital are two commonly used sedatives). Finally, aspirin is often used to treat a variety of ailments in dogs. Use the following guide for daily dosage: one tablet for every 20 pounds of the dog's weight, and no more than 2 tablets for dogs over 40 pounds; if you have baby aspirin, use one for every 10 pounds of weight (a maximum of 8 for large breeds, 6 for medium-sized dogs, and 4 for small ones).

*309. What about giving my dog human sedatives?*   This isn't a good idea at all. Sedatives should be given *only* under a veterinarian's supervision.

*310. How about giving my dog some of my diet pills?*   No. *Never.* This would drive the dog crazy with tension and anxiety—and could also be physically damaging.

*311. If our dog is sick, should we prepare a special area for her?*   Keep her comfortably warm (about 72°F. or 22°C.), off cold surfaces, and away from main traffic areas. Also, try to keep her isolated from other animals.

*312. My dog has been ill and hasn't eaten in several days. How can I get her to take some food?*   To hand feed a debilitated dog, elevate the animal's head, open her mouth, and spoon in a small portion of baby food or soup. Then close the mouth and hold it shut while the animal swallows. (Never force food on a dog that's spitting it out.) Another approach is to substitute broth or chicken soup for water. Most dogs will take water, even if they don't feel like eating, and if you offer soup instead this should help build back the animal's appetite and strength.

*313. Will a dog keep a wound clean by licking it?*   No. Allowing a dog to lick a wound in the belief that he's somehow cleaning it is actually harmful. The irritation from the constant licking causes increased inflammation, and since the dog's mouth

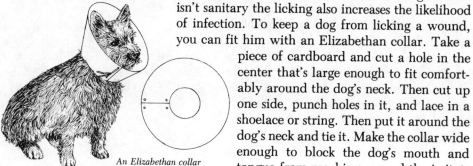

*An Elizabethan collar*

isn't sanitary the licking also increases the likelihood of infection. To keep a dog from licking a wound, you can fit him with an Elizabethan collar. Take a piece of cardboard and cut a hole in the center that's large enough to fit comfortably around the dog's neck. Then cut up one side, punch holes in it, and lace in a shoelace or string. Then put it around the dog's neck and tie it. Make the collar wide enough to block the dog's mouth and tongue from reaching around the irritated spot. The collar might annoy the dog a little, but it will allow his troubled skin some time to heal. An alternative to the cardboard collar is an old plastic bucket—cut a hole in the bottom and attach it the same way.

**314. My dog just had surgery. Is there anything I should do to make sure the stitches are all right?** When you get the animal home, look at the stitches. They should be tight, with the sides of the skin meeting cleanly in a smooth line. There should be no redness and no discharges immediately after surgery (315). If you don't see any abnormalities, leave the stitches alone—if you put something on them or worry over them too much you'll only call them to the animal's attention.

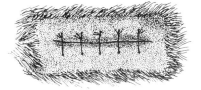

*A neat suture line*

**315. What signs of trouble should I look for after my dog undergoes surgery?** Although there shouldn't be any redness or discharges immediately after surgery, a small amount of redness and swelling around the suture line can be expected during the next few days. Sometimes there will also be a light drainage—this may be slightly bloody at first, but generally it should be clear. If the dog licks the incision, the swelling and redness are likely to increase, but it's no cause for alarm unless the licking is persistent. However, if the discharge becomes pus-like and foul-smelling and becomes heavier, and if the redness intensifies and spreads beyond the incision, the area could be infected. It should be examined by your vet within 24 hours.

Within about three days after surgery, a dog should show signs of regaining his strength and appetite. If the dog is vomiting persistently—say three or four times in six hours—two or three days after an operation, or if he's still moping around and not eating anything or drinking water after three days, you should have the animal re-examined by your vet. Another problem to watch for is a large swelling around the incision. If this happens, there may be an accumulation of fluid between the muscle tissue and the skin, or some of the internal stitches may have broken down and let the dog's internal organs come through, a condition known as evisceration. This is usually accompanied by listlessness, lack of appetite, vomiting, and occasional diarrhea. If you don't have this checked immediately, the dog's abdominal organs could protrude. This is *very* dangerous. The dog could go into shock and die within 12 hours.

**316. If the dog's stitches are itching, would it be all right to put baby powder on them?** No. This can cause an infection and keeps air from circulating over the incision.

**317. My dog is pulling at his stitches. How can I keep him from hurting himself?** If the dog is aggravating the condition of the incision, causing it to swell, redden, and give off a discharge, apply a mild antiseptic solution or even an antibiotic ointment. Antibiotic powder is also good because the powder helps to dry up the discharge while it's fighting the infection. If the dog has really tugged at the stitches and pulled some of them loose you should call your vet.

**318. Why don't veterinarians use absorbable stitches so that I'm saved the bother of coming back to have the nylon or metal ones removed?** Absorbable, or "gut," sutures can cause inflammation around the incision and this may interfere with healing and leave a scar. Another disadvantage is that the sutures may come out in three or four days if the dog licks them very much—and this could be disastrous for the dog. On the other hand, nylon, stainless steel, and other synthetic materials come out when the vet is ready to remove them. It's also a good idea to have a second look at any surgery. Your vet shouldn't charge for having the stitches removed, so all you're sacrificing is a little time—and I feel it's worth it.

## Spaying and Castration

*319. Is there some birth control method available for dogs besides irreversible surgery?* Yes. One is a pill that can be used three ways. It can be given continually to keep the dog out of heat. It can also be used on a short-term basis for a couple of months to keep a heat from coming on. You can also use it when heat occurs in order to prevent ovulation. However, this product can only be used for two successive heats; then you have to skip one. The second kind of birth control product is put in the dog's food to prevent pregnancy. At this time, there are no known side effects from these drugs, and they *can* be useful. For example, if you're unsure of whether or not you want to breed your dog, these drugs can give you time to make up your mind. However, I don't advise using them for longer than two heats. No matter what claims are made for any medication, it isn't wise to keep a dog on it for a lifetime if you don't intend to breed her. Spaying is much less drastic, it doesn't change the animal's temperament or physical characteristics, and it's cheaper in the long run.

*320. Do you recommend the abortion shot that's available for dogs?* Only as a last resort. This shot must be given within 48 hours of mating. It's an estrogen product, and it can have serious side effects. If you absolutely must, use it once, and then have the dog spayed if you can't control her mating habits.

*321. Aren't there intravaginal birth control devices available for dogs?* They've proven to be ineffective, costly to insert, and a bother for the dog.

*322. What is spaying?* Spaying is the removal of the ovaries and the uterus. It's also called an ovariohysterectomy.

*323. When is the best time to have my dog spayed?* For the best results, have your dog spayed before she's a year old (325, 326). This will insure her the most protection from developing mammary cancer.

*324. Couldn't you just tie the dog's fallopian tubes to prevent pregnancy?* Yes, it's possible, but with the ovaries still intact, the dog runs a much greater risk of contracting mammary cancer and uterine infections. And she'll still come into heat twice a year.

*325. Should you wait for a dog to have her first heat before having her spayed?* No. This idea has become just as widespread as the notion that spaying stunts a dog's development. Neither one is true at all. A dog's maturity rate is unaffected by spaying, as long as it's done after the dog is six months old.

**326. *Isn't it best to let a female dog have a litter before having her spayed? Won't her maternal instinct be frustrated otherwise?*** No. And there are some important health reasons for spaying early. If you waited for a dog to have a litter before spaying her, you wouldn't be able to do it before she was a year and a half old. But if you spay her before she's a year old, you wipe out almost all possibility of her getting mammary cancer, which is quite prevalent in female dogs. The dog's maternal instinct isn't increased or decreased by having a litter or not having one. The dog won't become neurotic if she never has a litter.

**327. *Will spaying make my dog get fat and lethargic and change her personality?*** No, but it *does* settle an animal down a little bit. They may become less active if they already have that tendency, but what happens often depends upon the owner —how often you take the dog out, how much play time you spend with her, and so forth. If you watch the dog's diet and exercise her properly there's no problem. The operation doesn't change the dog's personality.

**328. *Doesn't spaying rob a female dog of the joy of the sexual experience?*** The anthropomorphic idea that female dogs take the same pleasure from sex as human beings is not borne out by the reality of canine sexual interaction. The female's heat is a physiological phenomenon that occurs about twice a year for the purpose of having puppies. Allowing dogs to mate for their sexual pleasure is a misguided motive, particularly in the case of roaming males. It results in litter after litter of unwanted pups—a cruel and indefensible price to pay for pleasure that exists only in the mind of the dog's owner. Dog and cat populations are artificially sustained by society, with few natural checks. It's up to us to make sure they're responsibly controlled.

**329. *Should you only spay a dog between heats?*** It's best to spay a dog either between heats or three months after whelping. It *is* possible to spay a dog while she's in heat, but the uterus is enlarged at that time, and there's much more blood loss if spaying is performed then than if it's postponed. It's safer to spay the dog when she's two or three weeks pregnant than it is to do it while she's in heat. Probably the worst of all times to spay is when the dog is nursing. Spaying then would greatly reduce her milk production, and that could be very dangerous to the pups.

**330. *Why has there always been such emphasis on spaying females and so little talk about castrating males?*** As recently as ten years ago, it was almost taboo to castrate a male dog. This was no doubt connected to the fact that almost all veterinarians at the time were men. Owners have also had a prejudice against this practice; somehow they relate a roaming male dog to natural virility and they don't wish to interfere. The result is a population explosion of unwanted, starving, or destroyed puppies. The truth is that castration is safe, effective birth control. It's cheaper than spaying, and it causes no physical hardship to the dog. It's also safer surgically than spaying, particularly for an older dog. Neutering a male dog is a responsible act that has benefits for the owner and the community.

**331. *What's involved in castration, and how soon can it be done?*** Castration is the surgical removal of the testicles. The operation can be carried out with no problem after the dog is nine months old, or any time after that.

*332. What effect will castration have on my dog's behavior? Will it cause any physical problems?* The only adverse effect castration may cause is a tendency to slow down and gain weight, both of which may be overcome with exercise and proper diet. In some cases, the dog may become a little too docile; however, if he was causing problems before, this is more than a fair exchange. Roaming, aggressiveness, and inappropriate mounting can be cut by about 75 percent.

*333. How long will it take for the effects of castration to appear?* If you're castrating for behavior reasons, signs of change will begin to appear after about a month. Physically, the remaining sperm in the dog's reproductive system will be flushed out within about two days after castration.

*334. Would you recommend vasectomy as a birth control method for my dog?* Absolutely. If the dog hasn't got any personality problems that you want to change by having him castrated, a vasectomy is an excellent way of preventing unnecessary births.

PART IV

# BREEDING

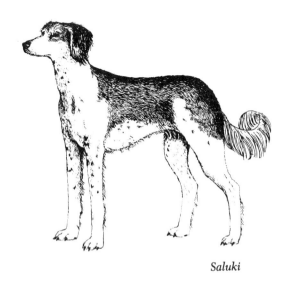

*Saluki*

Mating and Reproduction
335-359

Pregnancy and Birth
360-398

Caring for the Mother and Her Pups
399-431

Weaning
432-442

# Mating and Reproduction

**335. At what age do dogs become sexually mature?**   For males, sexual maturity arrives around the seventh to ninth month of age. A female will go into her first heat at different times, depending on the breed and the size of the dog. In general, small breeds have their first heat at six months, medium-sized dogs at around eight months, and large dogs between nine months and a year. However, some large breeds may not mature until as late as fifteen or sixteen months after birth.

**336. At what age do dogs lose their fertility?**   Normally, a female will stop going into heat around the age of twelve, or else the heats will become very irregular. Since very few people breed old dogs, not much is known about the late-life fertility of females. Males, however, are fertile as long as they live.

**337. What can be done about sterility? Can it be detected in advance?**   There's no practical way to know in advance of mating whether a dog will be sterile. Unsuccessful breeding attempts are the obvious evidence of this condition. Tests can then be done to determine the specific cause.

**338. When is a dog too old to have her first litter?**   This depends on the breed and the physical condition of the dog, but the maximum age is usually about seven years. However, if a dog hasn't had a litter by her third year, I'd suggest she be spayed. There's some danger in allowing an older dog to go through pregnancy because it puts a great strain on her body.

**339. How often will a female dog go into heat?**   The cycle occurs about twice a year. After the first heat, the cycles normally occur every six months, but some dogs may skip a heat. Irregular cycles generally involve missing a heat rather than having an extra one. It's very unusual for a dog to have more than two heats in a year.

**340. What exactly is the heat cycle?**   The changes undergone by a bitch in heat occur in four cyclic stages—proestrus, estrus, metestrus, and anestrus. Proestrus lasts about eight days, beginning when bleeding starts and the vulva shows signs of swelling, and ending when the female becomes willing to mate. During proestrus the female will attract males, but she'll be unwilling to copulate with them. Estrus is the period regarded as full heat. At this point the vaginal discharge reduces, the female accepts a male, and she ovulates. This fertile period lasts about four days. During metestrus, there are still signs of heat, but the vaginal discharge is reduced, the vulva regresses, and the female is no longer receptive to males. Metestrus lasts about five days. Anestrus designates the infertile period between heats, which usually extends about five and a half months.

**341. What are the signs that a female is coming into heat?**   The dog's vulva will swell up and then light bleeding will begin. This is called proestrus (340). When the dog is in full heat, the bleeding will stop. In most cases, the dog's personality remains much the same as it was before the heat, although she may be a little more nervous and active.

**342. *Should I breed my dog when she's in her first heat?*** No. The first heat signals the end of the maturation process, and if you breed a dog at this time her puppies may have congenital abnormalities. Another big disadvantage is the dog's emotional immaturity. She may be too upset by the experience of birth to be a good mother. There's also the danger of malnutrition for both the mother and her pups because her body is still demanding nutrients that will also be needed by her babies. For all these reasons, it's better to wait until the second heat.

**343. *Where's the best place to find a reputable stud? What should I look for in prospective candidates?*** Your best bet is to check with the local kennel club, the breeder from whom you bought your dog, or friends who have a dog like yours. Ask for references from past customers and examine the dog's pedigree papers. Talk to people who have used the dog in the past and find out if the puppies were healthy. Look for desirable traits in the dog—docility, good health, and intelligence. For larger dogs, especially German shepherds, there should be no evidence of hip dysplasia (602) and none in the dog's family history. Also consider the *size* of the dog. You don't want to mate a female with a dog more than 35% heavier than she is. A male that's larger than this will be more likely to produce puppies that are too large for the bitch, and she'll need a Caesarean section at the time of birth. Your preparations should begin three or four months before you expect your dog to go into heat so you have plenty of time to arrange the stud service.

**344. *What's the usual financial arrangement with the owner of a stud dog?*** Two methods of payment are common—a cash stud fee or first pick of one puppy out of the litter. On occasion, I've been asked about dividing a litter between the two parties, but I think this is unfair to the female dog's owner. After all, he or she spends much more time and money caring for the mother and her litter.

**345. *Is inbreeding dangerous?*** No, if it isn't done too extensively and doesn't perpetuate undesirable characteristics such as hip dysplasia, eyelid deformities, and other genetic defects and behavioral disorders. Certainly, if the choice is between a bitch's brother or father and a less desirable stud, the better dog is the best breeding choice.

**346. *How should I prepare my dog for breeding?*** Before she's mated, she should be worm-free and have all her shots. Both female *and* male dogs should be certifiably free of brucellosis (358).

**347. *When is the right time to get the stud and the bitch together?*** Wait until seven days after you see the first sign of bleeding and the first swelling of the vulva. If you want to be more exact, your vet can take a vaginal smear to pinpoint the day of full heat and ovulation. The smear should be taken around the sixth day of bleeding.

**348. *Will a bitch mate with a male before she's fertile?*** No. The female will resist any advances until she's in full estrus (340).

**349. *When they're mating, do dogs actually get stuck together so that they can't separate?*** Yes. The male's penis has a bone in it, and the muscle behind it swells up. In turn, the female has a muscle that clamps down, preventing the pair from separating until some time after ejaculation has occurred. The dogs may even turn around so that they're facing away from each other, but they can't break away until the mating response has run its course. The condition is known as copulatory lock, or the tie. When this happens, it's best to leave the two dogs alone. And it doesn't do any good to use the old folk cure of throwing cold water on them. They *can* be pulled apart, but it could cause damage to either or both dogs. This is a mechanical obstruction that will recede in ten or fifteen minutes, when the female relaxes. Any effort to separate the dogs forcefully will only create stress, and that will just prolong the tie.

**350. Is one mating enough, or should the dogs spend more time together?**  If the dogs breed on their first encounter, breed them again every two days up to a maximum of three times, or until the female will no longer accept the male. That should do it.

**351. What should we do if the dogs don't mate on the first day?**  Get them together every successive day until they do, and again two days after that. The dogs can stay together for the two days if it's convenient and they're getting along.

**352. Is it true an inexperienced stud dog may need some instruction on how to properly mount a female in heat?**  A dog that doesn't grow up in the wild and never sees other dogs mating may not know quite what to do, although he'll be eager to do *something*. It's occasionally necessary to go over and place the stud in the right position to mount the female. With any brains at all, he can take it from there.

**353. Are females in heat ever so coy that they never actually allow the male to mount?**  Some females may go into heat and never be completely willing to mate. At first, this could be due to inexperience, but if it continues, it's probably caused by a hormonal imbalance. The mating instinct is triggered by hormone changes; without the right chemistry, she won't be moved to complete the mating process.

**354. What can we do if the dogs never breed?**  The female can be artificially inseminated. There's less chance of pregnancy this way, but it may be worth the effort with a particularly valuable dog.

**355. Can a female in heat be impregnated by more than one male?**  Yes. If you're trying to breed a dog to a specific mate, keep her away from other males or you may get quite a mixed selection of puppies. If you buy a purebred dog with all his papers but he grows up looking a bit different from the standard of the breed, allow for some individuality. But if you're fairly sure that all is not what it seems, take some good pictures of the dog and send them to the American Kennel Club with a letter of explanation. They can advise you, and you may be able to get your money back.

**356. What forms of abortion are available for dogs?**  There's a kind of "morning-after" estrogen shot that can be used only in the first 48 hours after mating. However, there are problems with its use. This estrogen has been shown to cause cancer in humans, and it may not be safe for the dog. I feel it shouldn't be used more than once or twice on any individual dog. An alternative means of abortion is spaying, which can be done as late as the sixth week of pregnancy—in the first two trimesters. This is completely safe, and far better for the dog (319, 322).

*357. Do chlorophyll tablets affect a female in heat?*   Chlorophyll tablets reduce the attracting odor females give off during heat, but they don't provide any real security if you're trying to prevent or control pregnancy.

*358. Do dogs get venereal diseases?*   They don't suffer from the same ones that plague human beings, but they *do* have two of their own. One is called the transmissable venereal tumor, and it's caused by a virus which spreads through sexual contact. To guard against this, don't let your dog roam and breed indiscriminately, and have any potential partner checked for the virus by a veterinarian. Dogs also contract brucellosis, which is spread primarily by sexual contact and can be transmitted to humans. Brucellosis is a bacterial infection that attacks the genitals of dogs and is usually transmitted by vaginal discharges. However, infected blood, urine, semen, or milk can also carry it. Brucellosis can cause abortions in pregnant dogs. The disease produces no visible signs, so a blood test is necessary to confirm its presence. A dog usually only has to be tested once prior to breeding. After that, providing the animal's mating habits haven't been promiscuous, it's sufficient just to make sure that any future mates have been declared free of the disease.

*359. Is there any truth to the idea that once a purebred dog mates with a mongrel she's no longer capable of producing puppies that are purely her own breed?*   Absolutely not. She'll give birth to mutts as a result of *that* mating, but if she's bred to another purebred dog in the future, the pups will also be purebred.

## Pregnancy and Birth

*360. How can you tell when a dog is pregnant?*   A veterinarian can usually tell within the third or fourth week by palpating the dog's abdomen. During the fifth or sixth week, the abdomen swells noticeably and the dog's nipples enlarge.

*361. Do dogs have false pregnancies?*   Yes. This phenomenon occurs not long after a dog goes through a heat. The female will develop all the outward signs of pregnancy—her mammary glands will swell, she'll make preparations for whelping, and she may even adopt some small, furry object like a toy or a slipper and carry it around and mother it. The symptoms usually start two or three weeks after a heat and reach a peak in about six weeks. During this time, the dog may become reclusive and lose her appetite. Your veterinarian can give you drugs to break the cycle if the condition becomes too much trouble, but if false preganacy is a regular occurrence, you should consider having the dog spayed.

*362. After breeding, how long is it until the puppies are born?*   The gestation period for dogs is between 58 and 68 days, with the average being about 63 days. This is generally true regardless of the breed or the size of the dog.

*363. What's the best diet for a pregnant dog?*   Good nutrition is essential during pregnancy, and it's excellent preventive medicine for insuring healthy puppies. The most important change in the dog's diet while she's pregnant is the need for extra protein. Her requirement of protein will double, and her diet will have to be supplemented. You can add eggs to her usual meal, along with some powdered milk or cottage cheese, as well as additional dog food (70). Another crucial part of the mother's diet is calcium, particularly during the last four weeks of gestation.

**364.** *Will giving the dog plenty of supplemental calcium prevent her from having a calcium deficiency?* Not always. Be sure to give the dog extra vitamin D and calcium, such as powdered milk or bone meal, during the last four weeks of pregnancy so that her body has a chance to metabolize it completely.

**365.** *Should a pregnant dog get less exercise?* Her exercise should be cut back during the last three or four weeks of pregnancy, but this is something the dog will naturally do on her own. She can go about her daily activities, but she shouldn't be encouraged to do more than what's necessary.

**366.** *Is it all right to give a pregnant dog worm medicine?* Absolutely *not*. In fact, it's best not to give a pregnant dog *any* medication that hasn't been cleared with your veterinarian. Some wormers can be highly toxic to the fetuses.

**367.** *Does a pregnant dog need any special grooming?* Prior to whelping, it's a good idea to trim the hair away from the dog's nipples. This will make it easier for the puppies when they try to orient themselves, and easier for you to check on the condition of the breasts to watch for possible infections (404).

**368.** *What size litter can we expect?* It depends on the size of your dog. Small dogs usually have fewer puppies per litter. For instance, toy poodles ordinarily have only two or three pups at a time, while it's common for St. Bernards to have a litter of twelve puppies. The average, forty-pound dog will have six or seven pups.

**369.** *What kind of place should I prepare for the coming birth?* The dog will need a whelping box that has sides about 18″ high so the pups can't climb out. The space should be sufficient to hold both the mother and newborns comfortably, and it should be provided with some bedding. (Shredded paper is good, cheap, and easy to clean up. Remember to put several layers of *unshredded* paper underneath for cushioning and absorption.) If you have a small dog, you'll need to cut a door in the box so she can get in and out easily. The door can still have an edge on it that's from 3″ to 6″ high, depending on the size of the puppies. Larger dogs will need less of a door or none at all. About two weeks before whelping, get the dog acquainted with the box—feed her near the box, try to get her to sleep there; and if she's reluctant to sleep in the box in the place you've picked out for housing the brood, put the box in your bedroom for a while to help her feel at ease. The place where the puppies are born and reared should be one in which the dog will feel comfortable and secure. That's what the mother wants, and that's what you'd better plan for.

**370.** *What supplies will we need for the whelping?* Clean towels, dental floss, scissors, petroleum jelly, and an alum shaving pencil in case an umbilical cord happens to bleed after it's tied off and severed.

**371.** *My dog has gone several days past the date when she was due to give birth. What's wrong?* If the dog is a week overdue (362), there may be some problem, but three or four days is within the normal range, especially if she shows no signs of going into labor. If she *has* shown some of the preliminary signs (372) and then didn't follow this with whelping, she should be examined by your vet. Labor is triggered by hormonal stimulation given off by the fetuses. Sometimes when a dog has picked up a viral infection late in her pregnancy it can kill the litter. When this happens, the fetuses don't supply the proper hormones, and the mother fails to give birth.

**372. *How can I tell when my dog is ready to give birth?*** The day before whelping, a bitch will usually lose her appetite, a very noticeable change after weeks of eating extra portions to feed the fetuses. She'll become restless, and she'll go to the whelping box (or whatever location she's selected) and begin nesting moves—lying down and then getting up, circling, turning, digging, over and over again. This is the first stage of labor. Another signal is her temperature. About 24 hours before the birthing begins, her temperature will drop from a normal of 101° to 99°F. (38.3° to 37.2°C.). By taking the dog's temperature every day for four days prior to her estimated due date, you can pinpoint when the whelping will start and make your plans accordingly (297). Once the first stage of labor begins, the "water sac" containing the pups will break, and you can expect the dog to produce her first pup within the next twelve hours.

**373. *The labor pains have begun. When should the first pup emerge?*** During the second stage of labor, marked by abdominal contractions and panting, the dog will bear down and press to get the pups out. One should emerge within two hours after this heavy labor begins. If you don't see one after four hours, contact your vet (376).

**374. *When our dog is in labor, how much time should there be between the emergence of the puppies?*** After having a pup, the female will rest for anywhere from half an hour to two hours before going into labor again. There should be a break of no more than four hours between pups. One hour is about average.

**375. *What if the dog goes into heavy labor for a couple of hours and then quits?*** Several things could be wrong. This condition could be caused by dystocia, a malpresentation of the fetus; the pup could be breeched or be too large; or the dog could be suffering from uterine inertia, in which the muscles become fatigued and the animal just seems to give up. In any case, your vet should be called because the dog may need a Caesarean section or require drugs to stimulate the uterus.

**376. *When is a Caesarean section necessary? Does this make a dog sterile afterward?*** A Caesarean section is the surgical removal of the puppies from the uterus. By itself, a Caesarean section doesn't change the functioning of the dog's sexual organs or her ability to reproduce in the future. However, dogs are often spayed after a Caesarean section to prevent a recurrence of the problem that made the operation necessary in the first place. There are several conditions that may make a Caesarean section necessary, but the decision should be made by your veterinarian. The important thing for a dog owner to know is *when* the dog should be taken for medical help. In general, if a dog is in labor for more than four hours and produces no pups, or if she produces one and then no more during the next four hours, the animal should be taken to your veterinarian. Wait at least two hours, but no more than four. If there's obviously something wrong, and the puppies can't be delivered naturally, that's usually the point at which a Caesarean section becomes necessary. Once a dog has delivered two or three pups, the likelihood of problems with the rest of the litter is diminished.

**377. If my dog needed a Caesarean section delivery once, will she need another the next time she gives birth?**  For breeds that have large puppies and congenitally small birth canals and pelvises—such as the bulldog—Caesarean sections will be the only practical way of giving birth. However, if the dog was first mated with a larger male that gave her oversized puppies and then was mated with a smaller male, a Caesarean section may not be required.

**378. Are the puppies supposed to come out head first?**  Either head or rear first is normal.

**379. The first pup is out. Should we wait for the mother to break the sac that encases it?**  Each puppy emerges encased in a clear gelatinous material called the amniotic

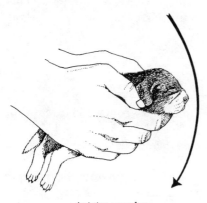

*Assisting a newborn*

sac. Normally, the mother will break this sac a minute after the pup is born. Then she'll lick and nuzzle the puppy to make him breathe; her licking will clean out the secretions. However, some dogs are very excited and confused when whelping, and they may not do this. Wait about a minute, and if the mother doesn't break the sac, pick up puppy and gently tear him free. Then grab the pup in both hands, holding his head up, and swing him in a small arc to throw the secretions out of his nose. You should also massage him gently to get him to breathe.

**380. Once a puppy is born, should we move him out of the whelping box while the next birth is taking place?**  Yes. The bitch will usually move around a lot between births, and she may accidentally step on a puppy. If the box is large, the newborn pups can be put to one side while the birthing continues. If there isn't enough space to accomodate them, using a second box is advisable. Be sure to wrap the pups in a towel to keep them warm.

**381. Everything seemed to be going well, and the pup started to emerge—but then he withdrew back inside. What can we do?**  Once a puppy has started to come out, he shouldn't withdraw. If this happens, get some petroleum jelly and spread it on the vulva. Then try to grasp the reluctant pup and extract him gently. *Don't* pull too hard, *don't* squeeze him. Just pull, firmly and

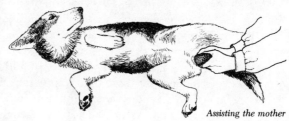

*Assisting the mother*

steadily, and if you feel resistance *don't* try to force the pup out. At this point, you should call your veterinarian for instructions.

**382. If the mother's vagina becomes dry during birthing, should it be artificially lubricated?**   Yes. If a puppy doesn't come out easily and if the vagina appears dry, you can apply some petroleum jelly.

**383. Is a long delay in the labor harmful to the pups that haven't been born yet?**   No, as long as the pup isn't partially out of the vulva and stuck. If this happens, you may need to help extract the puppy (381). But if the dog has stopped going into labor and you're fairly sure that there are more to be born, take her to your vet (375).

**384. How will we know when the last puppy has been born?**   It's very rare for a dog to retain a live pup in her uterus, but occasionally a dead puppy won't be expelled (371). This sometimes poses a problem because it's almost impossible to tell if there are still puppies inside by feeling the dog's abdomen. Of course, for a breed that has large litters, if the mother gives birth to two pups and then stops, you know right away that something's wrong. But for breeds that have small litters, the birth of two or three pups may seem quite normal. Because of this, and just as a good health precaution, it's a good idea to have the dog examined by your vet the day after she delivers. Your vet can give her a shot to contract her uterus, which will expel any remaining placentas. It's possible that the mother can abort the dead fetus later, but this isn't something to gamble on because it usually doesn't happen. Most of the time, when a dead pup isn't removed medically, the body remains in the uterus and decomposes, causing a bad uterine infection. Eventually, the mother's body will begin to reabsorb the puppy, and this can cause severe illness or death.

**385. Does the mother eat the afterbirth?**   About 15 minutes after each puppy is born a placenta will be expelled. The pup will still be attached to it by the umbilical cord. The mother will usually eat the placenta and chew off the umbilical cord.

**386. What becomes of the amniotic sac? Does the mother eat this too?**   The amniotic sac isn't much more than a bubble. When the mother licks the puppy, it will disintegrate.

**387. The dog hasn't cut the umbilical cord. Should we step in and do this for her?**   Give her fifteen or twenty minutes to cut the cord, and if she doesn't chew it off then you can clip it. It's wise to wait that long because there's blood in the placenta that the pup can use. By leaving the umbilical cord intact for about fifteen minutes after birth you'll enable that blood to flow into the puppy. After that, tie off the cord with dental floss (370) about two inches from the puppy. Make a second knot just past the first one, and cut in the middle.

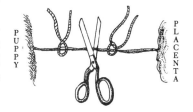

**388. Our dog cut the new puppy's umbilical cord with her teeth, but she hasn't eaten the placenta. Is there something wrong?**   No. The mother may not eat every placenta, particularly if there's a large litter, because it's just too much to eat and too much trouble. As long as she cut the umbilical cord, she's taking care of things. If she doesn't eat the placenta after fifteen or twenty minutes, you can dispose of it for her just to get it out of the way.

*389. Is there a danger that the mother dog will eat her puppies?* It's very unusual. This is more common with dogs in the wild. It's evidently a fear response in which the mother tries to hide the evidence of the birth when she feels threatened. The dog may also eat a badly malformed or dead pup. However, the usual response is simply to ignore such a pup. A well-domesticated dog giving birth to a litter in a secure environment is very unlikely to harm her pups.

*390. What causes a prolapsed uterus, and what can be done about it?* A prolapsed uterus protrudes from the body of the dog. In effect, it's been turned inside out by an excessive amount of straining. This is an *emergency* medical situation. Since it's outside the dog's body, the uterus will swell, and it may be cut off from the circulatory system. Try to keep the uterus as clean as possible and rush the dog to your veterinarian for help. There's *no* home remedy for this kind of problem. The longer the uterus is outside the dog's body, the more critical the situation becomes.

*391. Can a prolapsed vagina be treated at home?* The protrusion of the vagina can occur during heat or whelping. You can push it back into place (some sugar-water and ice applied to the vagina will reduce the swelling and make this easier), but your vet should also examine the dog and will probably suture the failing tissue to prevent the vagina from coming out again.

*392. If a puppy isn't breathing, is artificial respiration worth trying?* It's unusual for this to work, but it's certainly worth a try. Mouth-to-mouth resuscitation is easier to accomplish with a puppy because the animal's mouth can be sealed more completely (446). But don't blow in as hard as you would with a grown dog. If the puppy has just emerged, it will also be necessary to clear the nostrils by swinging the pup down in a small arc (379).

*393. Why are puppies born with their eyes closed?* Essentially, the pups are born prematurely. Both their eyes and their ears aren't fully developed at the time of birth. The shortened gestation period of dogs is probably a result of life in the wild in a roaming, pack environment—female dogs couldn't remain pregnant for long and still keep up with the other members of the pack.

*394. What kind of physical problems should I look for when I'm examining the newborn puppies?* You may want to have the pups checked by your vet for congenital abnormalities because some of these problems can be repaired easily when the pup is young. One of the most common birth defects is a cleft palate. This can be repaired surgically. It's also a good idea to examine the bone structure of the puppies. Short, thick-legged breeds such as bulldogs and Pekinese are particularly prone to a condition known as achondroplasia, or swimmer syndrome. The pup's legs point out to the side of the body instead of down, and he has to move about in a kind of crawl. There's no cure for this, and the pup is usually euthanized. Atresia anus is another rare but often fatal birth defect. A pup with this defect is born without an anus. Sometimes this can be corrected surgically, but the success of such an operation depends on how much tissue there is to work with.

*395. What can be done for a hydrocephalic puppy?* It's usually best just to euthanize the pup. Hydrocephalus, or water on the brain, is a particularly bad problem for the small breeds. The dog's cranium becomes filled with fluid, which prevents the bones of the head from sealing. Often this doesn't allow for the development of very much actual brain tissue.

**396. *Is it true that the mother will reject her puppies if people handle them?*** That isn't true—but you shouldn't take the puppies away from her and keep them for very long on the first day because this might interfere with the bond she's developing with them. However, you *can* handle them a bit; the mother won't mind.

**397. *Do male dogs have a paternal instinct toward their offspring?*** I've never seen any sign of it. If you were thinking of bringing Pop around to see the family, don't bother. It could be that this trait has been domesticated out of them.

**398. *We have two other dogs. Is it all right if they're around the mother and pups after they're born?*** This is a *bad* idea. You should keep other dogs away from the new family as a kind of precautionary quarantine. If other dogs live in the house, try to arrange separate quarters. This will protect all the animals from passing infections around and prevent possible fighting between the dogs. Mother dogs often become very defensive; they don't appreciate having other animals around their puppies.

## Caring for the Mother and Her Pups

**399. *What kind of diet should a mother dog have after the puppies are born?*** Maintain the same dietary supplements that you've been giving her during late pregnancy, emphasizing extra calcium for milk production. The food intake for the mother should stay high until the puppies are about four weeks old (432).

**400. *Is it true that the mother's milk helps immunize the puppies against certain diseases?*** It certainly does. That's why it's extremely important that the puppies all feed on the mother's milk during the first two days. If you have a weak puppy that's unable to feed well, you should force the milk into him. Squeeze some of it out into a little bottle and hand-feed him with an eyedropper (411).

**401. *How soon should the mother and puppies be examined by a veterinarian?*** This is usually done within the first week, especially if the pups' tails have to be docked or the dew claws need to be removed.

**402. *What kind of medical problems should I be concerned about with the mother?*** There are three major things to beware of: (1) uterine infection, (2) mastitis, an infected breast, and (3) eclampsia, or milk fever, a serious calcium deficiency.

**403. *There's a discharge coming from the dog's uterus, and the puppies were born a week ago. Is this a sign of infection?*** Some discharge will continue after birth for ten days to two weeks. The nature of the discharge will tell you if there's an infection or not. Normally, the flow should be reddish colored at first, and then become brown to light brown. If there's an infection, the discharge will contain mucus, be dark, and have a foul smell—and it will last longer than two weeks. This could mean the dog has retained a dead puppy or a placenta. Take her to your vet for an examination.

*404. How can you tell if a breast is infected?*   The dog's teat will look red and feel hot. The milk may be yellow, green, or red and have a pungent smell.

*405. What causes a mammary infection?*   Usually it's caused by a malfunction of the gland which keeps it from discharging properly. Eventually this causes an inflammation that in turn allows an infection to take hold.

*406. What kind of treatment is necessary for mastitis? Will it affect the puppies by contaminating the milk?*   If an infected mammary gland is treated with antibiotics, you'll probably have to hand-feed the puppies. If it is treated topically, your vet will probably bandage the teat, and you may have to milk out the gland and apply warm compresses to it. The rest of the time, keep it covered so the puppies don't have access to it.

*407. What can be done if the mother dog doesn't have enough milk?*   If the mother is getting plenty of dietary supplementation, but her milk production is still low, the pups may have to be hand-fed (411). To judge whether the amount of milk is sufficient, express each nipple. If only two or even four of them produce milk, and if the pups are feeding all the time but not getting anything to eat, you'll have to step in to prevent health problems. An alternative to hand-feeding may be to find a surrogate mother—a healthy, good-sized dog that just had a small litter (two or three pups), or whose pups are just being weaned.

*408. What are the signs of eclampsia?*   The mother dog will have tremors, she'll become weak and suffer from chills, and she'll have a lower than normal body temperature (288). Her heartbeat will also be irregular. If the condition reaches the advanced stages, she'll go into convulsions and she may die. Eclampsia usually arises about two weeks after birth if the dog isn't getting enough calcium to support herself and the puppies. *This is an emergency situation.* The dog's heart requires calcium in order to keep pumping properly, and the dog can die within four to six hours after the symptoms first appear. If the dog begins to appear weak and starts trembling, keep the puppies away and take her to your vet. Letting the puppies continue to feed will make the condition much worse.

*409. Is something wrong with a mother dog whose coat is shedding and becoming very thin?*   This is a common occurrence during pregnancy and for about three months afterward. The dog's protein is being used to sustain the puppies instead of to maintain her coat. Her coat should recover its normal thickness within three months, and its condition can be helped until then with dietary supplements (108).

*410. How do you care for an orphaned litter of pups?*   Keep the room temperature around 80°F. (26.6°C.) and hand-feed (411) the puppies small meals six times a day for the first two weeks, then four times after that until they're weaned. Be careful not to overfeed the pups, and weigh them daily to make sure they're growing and getting enough to eat. When they're three weeks old, you can start mixing some baby cereal with their formula in preparation for weaning (432).

*411. How do I hand-feed a puppy?*   This has to be done with a puppy-feeding kit, an eyedropper, or a little doll-sized baby bottle; be sure *not* to use a glass eyedropper. There are commercial formulas available for puppies, and the labels will give you directions on the quantities to use for the size of your puppy. Consult with your veterinarian on how to prepare a home-made formula and how much to feed the pups (410).

**412. Is there a runt in every litter?** No. Some litters are composed of uniformly healthy and normal-sized pups. The term "runt" is a colloquial expression with a vague meaning. Some people use it to designate the smallest puppy, even though this one may be the healthiest of the lot, while others call a sickly pup a "runt." The expression is so ambiguous that it's almost meaningless.

**413. What kinds of diseases can I watch for that may affect our new puppies?** Two viruses—corona virus and parvovirus—frequently attack puppies when they're four to six weeks old. These viruses cause vomiting and severe, bloody diarrhea. They're mostly a problem in kennels, where they're transmitted from puppy to puppy; they rarely occur in litters born at home. If a pup shows signs of having a virus, get the animal to your vet as fast as you can. Until you can get the pup to a vet, keep him away from the mother and siblings. Feed the affected pup cottage cheese and baby cereals to counteract the diarrhea, and increase his intake of fluids by hand-feeding (411). Give him vitamin supplements, especially B and C, and sugar-water (a teaspoon of sugar to eight ounces of water) to provide enough glucose for quick energy.

**414. What are some of the diseases that the puppies can get from contact with other dogs?** When puppies die at an early age, there are usually so few traceable causes that it's difficult to point to a particular illness. It's a situation similar to crib death in human infants. However, the herpes virus is one of several that are usually responsible. There's no treatment for pups that have been affected by the herpes virus, and there's little or no warning before death occurs. Adult dogs rarely contract herpes virus, and when they do it usually runs its course, but they can remain carriers for other people. Distemper and tracheobronchitis are two other communicable diseases that young pups could pick up, although the odds that they'll contract these infections are not as likely as the risk of contracting herpes virus.

**415. The umbilicus of one of our puppies has become very sore and red. Can this be treated at home?** Yes. Put some mild antiseptic solution on a clean rag and hold it against the pup's umbilicus for a few minutes twice a day. A bad infection may need to be treated with antibiotics, but normally this problem isn't that serious. Keep an eye on the pup to make sure the infection isn't spreading. If she seems to be increasingly lethargic, take her to your vet. This kind of infection can usually be prevented by making sure the bitch whelps in a clean place, and then keeping the area free of feces, urine, and dirt (419).

**416. What's wrong with a puppy whose belly button is popped out abnormally?** Sometimes the umbilicus never closes off completely; instead, it just seals over with a layer of skin. When this happens, fat, or even intestinal material, can protrude. This is called an umbilical hernia. Small protrusions can be ignored, but if the hernia is larger (about the width of your little finger), it may need surgical correction.

**417. What would cause some tissue to protrude from puppy's rectum, and what can I do about it?** This is likely to be a prolapsed rectum. It's mostly a problem for puppies under eight weeks old, who sometimes strain so hard to defecate that they break down the muscles around the rectal wall. This causes the wall to be squeezed inside out so that it protrudes from the animal's body. Once outside the body, the tissue will begin to devitalize, so you may need to replace it temporarily if the vet's office isn't nearby. Put ice in a washrag and hold it to the prolapsed tissue to help shrink it. Soaking the tissue with sugar-water will also help it to recede because this takes out some of the excess fluid. Next, lubricate the end of your finger with petroleum jelly and gently push the tissue back into place. Then take the pup to your vet.

**418. Do pups need heartworm preventive medicine?**   Until puppies are about eight weeks old, they're usually sheltered from mosquitoes because they spend their time inside. After eight weeks of age, they probably need to start heartworm medication if you live in an area where the worms are endemic. Ask your vet about this.

**419. Does the mother dog eat the puppy's feces?**   Yes. It seems to be a simple solution worked out by dogs for keeping the den clean. It's natural and harmless.

**420. Sometimes the mother dog will take a puppy's mouth and nose in her own and hold it shut. Why does she do this?**   This is one of her techniques for putting the puppy in his place. Watch the way the mother controls her puppies and you'll be able to use these same techniques later to discipline and train the puppy. The mother may pick a puppy up by the scruff of the neck and shake him, she may hold his snout shut, and she may use direct, eye-to-eye contact. This last method is something to remember if you encounter a stray dog. A lot of dogs will take it as a threatening gesture if you stare them in the eye.

**421. What can be done if the mother seems hostile to the puppies?**   This happens occasionally, especially if the bitch is nervous or hyperactive. It's more common with small breeds. This kind of mood will usually pass after the newness of the situation wears off. Spend some time with her and the puppies to reinforce the connection between them. If she ignores them and leaves the whelping box for long periods, take her back and stay with them for a little while. If she refuses to care for the puppies, you will have to either hand-feed them or find a surrogate mother (410). You should also consider spaying the dog because her temperament is obviously not suited for breeding.

**422. Will a mother dog pick out favorites in the litter and neglect others?**   Yes. The mother will usually pay less attention to the weakest puppies and devote more time and energy to the ones that are more assertive.

**423. One of the puppies in our litter is very weak, and the mother doesn't seem to take much interest in it. Should we try to nurse it ourselves?**   This situation is very common. Some puppies don't do well right from the start; often one puppy in a litter will weaken and eventually die. The mother's lack of response is a natural way of weeding out the weakest of her species, an automatic inbred behavior. A mother dog doesn't have the understanding to worry about every puppy, and her priorities are different from yours. If you want to try and revive the straggler, it *can* be worth the effort. Hand-feed it (411) and try to keep it warm. More attention and outside feeding can sometimes make the difference, but don't expect miracles.

*424. Will handling puppies too much make them sick?*  No. In fact, when they're from four to six weeks old they should be handled quite frequently to get them used to human contact. When they're younger than this, you can still play with them, but you shouldn't spend *too* much time with them because the mother will tend to cut back on caring for them if she sees you giving them a lot of attention. You should also remember not to neglect the mother. After a couple of weeks of nursing a litter of demanding little puppies, she may start to get bored, so it's a good idea to give *her* some attention at this point. She'll appreciate it.

*425. What is puppy stressing?*  It's a training process that involves getting the pups used to being handled. This pays off later when you have to give the adult dog a pill or shot, take his temperature, or clip his nails—any of the things that dogs struggle against. You can start puppy stressing when the pups are about three weeks old. It involves gently turning the pup upside down, handling him a lot, playing with his feet, gently opening and closing his mouth. All this is done playfully so that the pup gets used to the idea of being quite "man-handled." It's especially important to concentrate on positional changes (turning the pup, putting him on his back, and so forth) because getting the pup used to this kind of handling can make things a lot easier later in life. Since it's most effective between the ages of three to six weeks, puppy stressing is basically the responsibility of the person raising the litter. However, a new dog owner can carry this on in later weeks, and it can only help.

*426. When do a puppy's eyes and ears open?*  This usually happens around ten days to two weeks after birth. During this time, the external ear canal will open up and the outer ear will take shape.

*427. The pups' eyes are starting to open. What kinds of trouble should we be looking for?*  Normally a puppy's eyes open slowly over one or two days—they go from little slits to completely open eyes, as if the pup was doing a slow blink. If his eyes are still closed after he's 2 weeks old, or if they're only opening on one side and seem stuck and infected, have your vet look the pup over. If one of the pups develops a minor infection after his eyes open, you can wash the eye with warm water two or three times a day for a couple of days. If this doesn't clear up the infection, check with your vet.

*428. How well can the puppies see when their eyes first open?*  Their eyesight is very poor on the first day that their eyes open. Take care to keep them out of direct light and sunlight until they've had a couple of days to adjust to vision and learn to control their eyes and focus them.

*429. Our new puppies all have blue eyes. Will they stay that color?*  Puppies start out with blue eyes, but they change color after about a month. The permanent color of the eye may be blue or some other shade. The most common is brown.

*430. What's the best time to have the pups' tails docked?*  This can be done very easily at five days of age. There's little bleeding, and the process is medically simple.

*431. When should the puppies start leaving the whelping box?*  After two weeks, take them out and let them explore a bit. In another two weeks, they'll usually have outgrown the box. At this point, it's a good idea to prepare a larger enclosed area for them. Cover it with several layers of newspapers so that you can easily keep it clean. This will provide a secure den from which you can supervise their explorations.

## Weaning

**432. How soon should the puppies be weaned?** Start weaning them when they're about four weeks old. Begin by cutting back on the mother's food and vitamin supplements by about 50% for three to five days to reduce her milk production. Then bring the ration back up to the amount the dog was eating before she was bred. Also, offer the puppies milk formula and baby cereal as a substitute.

**433. Should the mother be present while I'm offering the puppies the formula and cereal?** No. Feed them when she's being walked or is away for some other reason. This way you won't have to worry about her eating their food. Remember, at the same time that the pups are learning to eat dog food, you're reducing the mother's ration in order to dry up her milk glands. This leaves her a little bit hungry.

**434. How can I teach the puppies what the food is and how to eat it?** You can introduce the food to the puppies by getting a little bit on your finger and touching it to their lips. Then show them the bowl.

**435. What about giving the pups ground meat while they're being weaned?** Ground meat can be used to help make the transition to dog food because it's softer and easier to digest. It helps the pups become accustomed to eating solid food. Boiling it a little bit will help make it easier on their digestion. You can start feeding small amounts of ground meat by hand during the first week of weaning, when the pups are four weeks old. At the same time, you'll be introducing them to eating out of a bowl with the formula and cereal mix. After a while, you can phase out the hand feeding of these bits of meat, as the pups move on to eating regular dog food.

**436. What about dunking the puppies' noses in the bowl? I've heard this is a good way to show them how to eat.** I think this is a bad idea because it can frighten the puppies unnecessarily. With a little more patience, they'll learn just as much, and without the possibility of getting milk up their noses and being scared.

**437. How many bowls should I use to feed the puppies?** Make sure that everybody is eating, but encourage a little competition. To do this, put down one bowl for every four or five puppies. A little shoving for the food will help make them less picky about food later on in life.

**438. How often should the puppies be offered a bowl of food?** Give the pups a bowl of formula and cereal a couple of times a day for the first three or four days. They'll still be feeding off their mother regularly at that point. When they start to take to eating on their own, give them three meals a day.

**439. The weakest pup of the litter has a lot of trouble getting up to the bowl to eat, and I think sometimes he gets very little. Should I feed him separately?** If the weak one isn't getting anything then you should feed him alone. However, try not to make a habit of this. Each time, wait and see if he'll force himself up to the bowl to eat. You don't want to encourage dependence and fearful behavior.

**440. When do I introduce the puppies to dog food?** When the pups are eating three meals a day from the bowl and are growing more accustomed to this schedule, add a little bit of dry dog food to one of the formula meals. The sooner they begin to eat dog food the better. It should be a part of their taste and eating habits as early in their lives as possible; at the same time, it's important to keep up their interest in eating from a bowl. To do this, gradually increase the amount of dry food in the bowl over the course of about ten days.

**441. How soon should the puppies be completely weaned?** When they're six weeks old, the puppies should be totally weaned away from their mother's milk. By this time, they'll be eating dry meal that's been moistened with milk three times a day. The meal should be a specific formula made for puppies. You can start introducing canned food to the puppies between the sixth and eighth weeks. By the time they're eight weeks old, they should also be eating dry meal that's moistened with water instead of milk.

**442. Is it a good idea to supplement the diet of puppies that have recently been weaned to dog food?** Yes. You can give the pups cottage cheese and eggs. If you're feeding them three times a day, give them an egg in the morning with their breakfast. They can also make good use of vitamin and mineral supplements, as well as brewer's yeast, which contains B vitamins.

# PART V

# ACCIDENTS AND AILMENTS

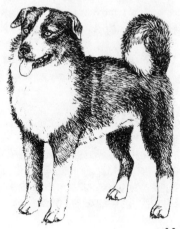

*Mutt*

### First Aid
443-494

### Common Ailments: Vomiting, Diarrhea, Constipation
495-500

### Eye, Ear, and Mouth Problems
501-516

### Respiratory Ailments
517-525

### Skin Conditions, Abscesses, Sores
526-535

### Muscle and Bone Problems
536-546

### External Parasites
547-570

### Internal Parasites
571-595

### Miscellaneous Ailments
596-600

# First Aid

***443. Is it all right to move a dog that's been struck by a car?*** Yes. Definitely. It's important both for your safety *and* that of the dog to get out of the road. If possible, the dog should be moved gently and supported from underneath (452,473) but in a dangerous situation, just grab the animal and drag him to safety. If the dog is in great pain, or if he's a strange dog, he may try to bite you, so tie a piece of rope or cloth around his muzzle as a precaution (457).

***444. Once the dog has been moved, what injuries should I look for first?*** Check for obvious external injuries—bad bleeding, cut limbs, and so forth. Wrap the injured areas tightly in a piece of cloth and apply pressure to stop the bleeding. The bandage should be as clean as possible, but it doesn't have to be sterile; if there's any infection, it's already in the wound. The important thing is to stop the bleeding (465).

***445. How can you tell whether a dog is dead? Unconscious?*** First check the blink response of the dog's eye. Unless he's dead or in a coma, the dog should blink when you touch the surface of the eye. You can also check for a heartbeat by feeling on the left side of the chest between the fifth and seventh ribs, pressing hard. Try for the animal's pulse if you can't be sure of the heartbeat (298). Also check the mouth—the most obvious sign is respiration, but the dog's gums provide clues as well (448).

***446. What should I do if the dog is having difficulty breathing?*** This is an indication that there may be lung damage. If the dog's tongue is turning blue, this is also a sign of respiratory distress. Until you can get the dog to a veterinarian, you can try emergency mouth-to-mouth resuscitation: cup the dog's mouth in your hands and blow through your mouth into his. You won't be able to blow through the nose if there's any major damage because the air passage will probably be clogged with blood. Do not attempt to breathe for the dog if his respirations are rapid but he is still turning blue. This is usually a sign that he has a hole in his chest; instead, locate the hole and cover it until you can get the dog to the vet.

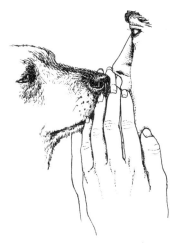

*Giving mouth-to-mouth resuscitation*

***447. How can I tell if there's internal bleeding?*** Check the color of the dog's gums. Some dogs have pigmented, black gums, so this won't work for them, but if the gums are normally pink, look for pale white or yellowish discoloration. However, if the bleeding is less severe or has just begun, the dog's gums may still have a healthy color. If you push your finger against the dog's gums, the pressure will make the gum turn white, but if there's normal blood flow and pressure it should only take one or two seconds for the gums to become pink again. If the gums stay white for a long time, you know the dog has had a drop in blood pressure or is losing blood somehow.

**448. Is it possible to give a dog heart massage?**   Yes, but this is only really useful in cases of electric shock (480). In an auto accident, the dog's heart failure is nearly always caused by a fatal loss of blood, and heart massage won't help. To give a dog heart massage, lay the animal on his side on a flat, firm surface. Place your hands on his chest and compress it firmly and quickly, pressing about 60 or 70 times a minute. Combine this with mouth-to-mouth resuscitation at a rate of about 10 breaths every minute (446). Gauge the force of your massage to the size of the dog. With very small dogs, heart massage can be accomplished by just squeezing the chest between your palms. If the dog is tiny, you can even do it in one hand. Don't worry about damaging the dog's ribs; they can heal—but they *won't* if his heart doesn't start again. If you see that pressing on the chest isn't working, pound firmly on the left

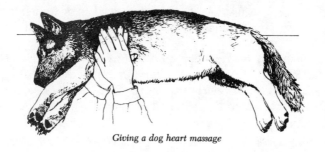

*Giving a dog heart massage*

side between the fifth and seventh ribs. The heart is a well-protected organ, and compressing it without surgically opening the chest cavity isn't easy. Fortunately, many dogs have narrow chests, and this increases the chances for effective heart massage.

**449. Is there a way to slow down an excessively fast heart rate?**   Put gentle pressure on the dog's eyes by pushing your fingers against his eyelids. This stimulates the vagus nerve, which will then cause the heart to slow down.

**450. A dog has been run over. She isn't bleeding, but she can't walk and seems to be in really bad shape. Should we have her put out of her misery?**   Don't be so hasty. Right after an accident, a dog's condition sometimes seems a lot worse than it really is. It can take a long time to get over the shock of being knocked down by a car, and the dog may just be stunned. Head injuries often swell up and look awful, but they can clear up quickly with a little attention. If the dog can't stand, you may think that her back is broken, but she may actually have a broken pelvis, which isn't a life-threatening injury. Check the animal over and give her time to recuperate before you decide that her condition is hopeless.

**451. Do dogs suffer from the same kind of medical "shock" that people get after a bad accident or injury?**   This kind of shock is the result of internal injury, and it affects dogs just as it does people. The major treatment is to administer intravenous fluids, often an impractical measure in a first-aid situation. However, the loss of fluids *does* make the dog get very cold, so try to keep the animal warm if you can (447).

**452. What's the best way to carry a dog?**   First, make sure that the animal hasn't broken any bones (472,473); once you're sure of this, you can pick up the dog. A small dog can be cradled in the bend of your arm, with your hand cupped across the animal's chest. For a slightly larger dog, grip the back of the rear legs with one arm and the front of the forelegs with the other. If the animal seems too large for this

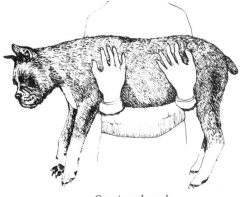

*Carrying a large dog*

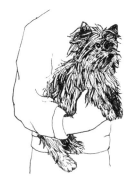

*Cradling a small dog*

kind of carry to be practical, hold the animal just inside each set of legs, with one arm on the chest and the other on the stomach. Don't try to pick up a very large dog alone. They're not dead weight, and a squirm from the animal can give you a serious back injury. It's much wiser to get help: have one person encircle the front legs and the other lock his hands around the rear legs; then both of you should lift together. When you're lifting a puppy, be sure to support his hind end so that he feels secure (14).

**453. How can I examine my dog to find out what's wrong with him when he cries every time I touch him? I know he's hurt, but I can't tell where.** With acute pain, there will be an obvious scream if you touch the sore spot. Unfortunately, dogs react to an injury by becoming hypersensitive to being handled. The dog gives out a yelp whenever he's touched. When this happens, let the animal sit until he grows calmer. Then work gently, reassuring the animal as much as you can.

**454. My dog was struck by a car. He's walking around, apparently just a little bit shaken up. What signs of trouble should I look for?** Many dogs seem all right at first, but later they reveal problems that are less obvious than a cut or a broken bone, but just as serious. If the animal seems okay, let him cool down for a little while. Then examine him thoroughly and treat any abrasions and scrapes that aren't too bad (469). If the dog is able to walk on all four legs you can be reasonably sure that there are no *broken bones* (472), but if he's weak and unstable on his back legs, there may be a pelvic fracture, a very common injury in automobile accidents (473). Also check to make sure the dog can urinate. Symptons of a *ruptured bladder* (lethargy, vomiting, and pallor) won't show up for another 48 hours, but by then it can be too late. If the dog hasn't urinated in 24 hours, get help right away. Also watch for a cough to develop a couple of days after the accident. This could indicate *lung damage*. See if the dog has difficulty eating, and check his teeth for cracks and breaks. Both are indications of a *fractured jaw*. Severe vomiting combined with respiratory and abdominal distress could mean that the dog has a *diaphragmatic hernia*, a tear in the diaphragm. When any of these signs occurs, a trip to your vet is in order.

**455. My dog was in an accident and is still having trouble breathing several hours later. What's wrong?** If you notice an extreme shortness of breath—a shallow panting—that persists several hours after the accident, this can mean that a puncture wound through the chest wall is causing a lung to collapse. This condition is easily treatable, but it must be looked after *soon*—it will become more serious if it's allowed to go unattended. Take the dog to your veterinarian immediately.

**456. Is there a safe way to stop a dog fight?** Don't rush in and try to pull the dogs apart—you'll be taking a chance because dogs aren't good at distinguishing between their opponent and an innocent bystander. Instead, make a loud noise, scream, throw water on them—do anything you can to distract them. In an extreme emergency, you may have to step in to save a little dog; but first you might want to try and grab the big dog by the collar. Either way, use a *lot* of discretion.

**457. Is there some quick way to subdue a vicious dog?** Make a muzzle out of a piece of rope or cloth about three feet long. With someone holding the dog's head from behind, wrap the rope up from under the chin and over the nose, securing it with a

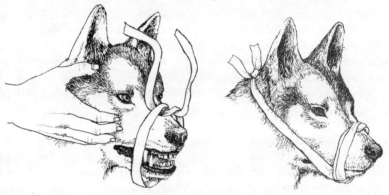

*Applying a makeshift muzzle*

loop—like the first step in tying your shoe. Then wrap the rope back down for a second half-knot under the chin. Finally, tie the ends of the rope behind the dog's head. If you're in a big hurry with a very nasty dog, use a wet piece of gauze or cloth and tie it over the dog's nose; the wetness will keep the cloth from slipping.

**458. What should you do when someone is bitten by a dog?** If the dog is a stray, call the city dog pound so they can capture the animal and keep him penned up until you can find out more about him. If the dog lives in the neighborhood, try to locate the owner and find out if the animal has had his rabies shots (616). Even if the dog wasn't rabid, you'll have to treat the wound with care. Dog bites invariably become infected, so the injured person should be treated by a doctor.

**459. My dog was in a fight and got bitten in a couple of places. Can I treat these wounds at home?** In most cases you can, but if the dog is bleeding badly or the wound is extensive, don't try to take care of it yourself—it could lead to a serious infection. Flush out the wound with soap and water, then apply hydrogen peroxide or another mild antiseptic solution (296). Really wash it well, and if it's a large wound, get the garden hose and keep it running on the wound for 10 minutes or longer.

Then you can treat the wound with antibiotic ointment, applied twice a day. If you notice that the wound is getting worse and the dog becomes feverish or lethargic, have the bite examined by your vet. A final word of caution: Some dog bites look small on the surface, but the skin has been ripped away from the connective tissue underneath. If the wound seems to open into a pocket under the skin, take the dog to your vet for antibiotic treatment.

*460. What causes heat stroke?* Heat stroke results when a dog is unable to eliminate body heat fast enough to keep his temperature down to a safe level. The only way dogs can control their body temperature is by panting, expiring internal heat through their breath. It's important for a dog to have access to a cool spot and plenty of water on hot days. A dog that's been chained up in the sun with no water, or left in a closed, hot car is an animal whose life is in danger.

*461. How dangerous is heat stroke?* Heat stroke that goes unattended for over 30 minutes can be fatal. If the dog doesn't die, there still can be brain damage.

*462. What are the signs of heat stroke? What should I do when my dog is suffering from them?* The dog will be extremely lethargic and will pant rapidly. If his gums are unpigmented, they'll be pale. The pupils of his eyes will be dilated, and his temperature will be about 105 to 107° F. (40.5 to 41.6°C.). When you see these symptoms, immediately cool the dog off as much as possible—turn on the hose or throw the dog in a bathtub full of cold water; even put ice in the tub. Continue this cooling for 10 or 15 minutes, then take the dog's temperature (297). Keep cooling the dog until his temperature is down to 103° F. (39.4° C.). Also give the dog aspirin (308). Once the dog has recovered and rested, watch him for signs of brain damage, such as dizziness, lack of coordination, and abnormal behavior.

*463. My dog is choking. What can I do?* Dogs choke most frequently on toys, food, and bones. A choking dog will be in obvious distress. Open his mouth and stick your thumb on the roof of it; this technique will force him to keep it open. Look down his throat and try to see if anything is stuck there (it helps to use a flashlight). If you find something, hold the dog's mouth open, reach in, and pull out the object. (You may need someone else's help to do this.) If the object remains stuck, try pulling the dog's tongue forward. This will lift the larynx up, and sometimes whatever's causing the blockage will just fall out. A dog's tongue is slippery, so use a cloth to get a grip on it. If you can't see anything but you really think something's stuck in the dog's

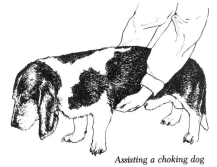

*Assisting a choking dog*

throat, it's time for a canine version of the Heimlich® maneuver. Get behind the dog, bend over him, place your hands together under his body, and pull up on the rib cage. This compresses the diaphragm, and should expel the object. If this fails, get the dog to your vet immediately. NOTE: if the dog is able to swallow food and water, he doesn't have anything stuck in his throat. Some dogs cough so harshly that it gives the impression they're choking.

**464. I think my dog has swallowed something. What should I do?**   Take the dog to your veterinarian because the treatment depends on what kind of object was swallowed. Some things may pass through the dog's system without a problem, providing they aren't sharp or rough. If they're small enough and you didn't witness the swallowing, you might never know anything strange had gotten into the dog's digestive tract. But if the object is large, it will block the dog's system and cause constant vomiting and bowel impaction. The dog will become extremely listless, and he'll have a tender abdomen and a fever. If the animal's digestion isn't blocked (if, for instance, he's swallowed a pin), then the symptoms are more vague and mild. Look for occasional vomiting and a lack of appetite. Remember, your veterinarian should be called to treat *anything* that will not pass through the dog's system.

**465. My dog stepped on something and cut his foot, and now he's bleeding a lot. What can I do?**   Paw cuts usually bleed a lot. First look at the dog's foot and see if there's anything stuck there. If so, get it out and then apply a pressure bandage to the foot for three or four hours. A pressure bandage is a tight binding designed to contain a badly bleeding wound *without* shutting off the circulation. To make one, you ought to have cotton, gauze, and adhesive tape, but in an emergency the gauze is optional —and if nothing else is available, a t-shirt and a belt can be turned into a workable pressure bandage. Begin by padding the wounded area thoroughly. In the case of a leg wound, circle the leg with about an inch of cotton and then cover it with a tight layer of gauze, about three wrappings. Once this is secured with a double layer of tape the bleeding should be controlled. This kind of emergency measure should *not* be left on the dog for more than 12 hours. When you remove the bandage, if you find that the bleeding has been stopped, flush out the wound with lots of water, antiseptic solution, and soap and put on a clean bandage. However, if the bandage keeps the bleeding in check only when it's on and the flow starts as soon as it's removed, put the bandage back on and take the dog to your vet. If the bandage fails completely to control the bleeding, you'll need to apply a tourniquet.

**466. How do you apply a tourniquet?**   The only places where a tourniquet is practical are the dog's legs and tail. Tie on a rope or a piece of gauze—above the elbow

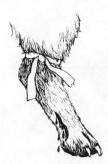 on the front leg or below the knee on the hind leg, depending on where the wound is. Make it tight enough to stop the bleeding or greatly reduce it. A tourniquet cannot safely be left on a limb for more than 30 minutes, but this gives you time to get the dog to a veterinarian or apply a firm pressure bandage to control the bleeding without stopping the circulation. In the past, there have been a number of theories about whether or not a tourniquet should be loosened periodically. To be safe, you should put it on and leave it alone until the wound is bandaged properly.

**467. Suppose a dog has a bad cut and you can't get to a vet for a long time. Should you try to stitch him up yourself with some sterilized thread?**   No. This will very likely introduce an infection into an already bad wound. Besides, I'm not sure any dog would stand still for this. The most important thing you can do is just stop the bleeding, flush the wound thoroughly with water, and put a firm bandage on the cut until you can get help (465).

**468.** *How do you decide if a cut needs stitches?* If a cut is to be stitched, it must be done within 24 hours or it will be difficult for it to heal. When stitching is used properly it can cut the wound's healing time in half. When I'm deciding whether or not to use stitches, I look to see if the cut is completely through the skin, to the point where the muscle tissue is visible below. If a cut is even deeper and there's a possibility that a tendon has been cut, then the wound automatically requires suturing. And if a cut is more than an inch long it should also be stitched.

**469.** *My dog has some minor scrapes and abrasions. What's the best way to treat them?* Wash the scrapes well with soap and water, swab them with an antibiotic solution, and then apply an antibiotic powder or ointment. If the dog insists on licking the scrapes, you can construct an Elizabethan collar (313).

**470.** *What could cause a dog to start limping all of a sudden? His foot isn't cut, and there isn't a thorn in it.* Watch the way the dog walks. If he's limping, but still putting weight on the leg, he probably has a sprain. Check for pain by squeezing the dog's leg a little bit to see how he reacts. If there's no increased sign of pain when you touch him, he probably has a strained tendon, ligament, or muscle. To treat this, give the dog an aspirin every six hours (308). Then let the dog rest. There should be a noticeable improvement in 24 hours. After this, be sure to take it easy. Don't run the dog. Walk him on a leash, and allow only minimal exercise for about 4 days.

If the dog yelps in pain when you touch his leg on the sore spot, but he's still putting weight on it, he has a sprained joint (453). Follow the same treatment procedure and keep the dog still. Watch him carefully, and if there's a lot of pain and soreness the next day, take the animal to your vet. Another possibility is that the joint is infected, something that can occur as a result of a penetrating wound like a bite. Any time you find a swollen joint, take the animal to your vet. The infection will only get worse the longer it goes unattended.

**471.** *What should I do if the dog never lets the leg touch the ground and cries when I touch it?* This is an indication of either a fracture (472) or a serious tendon or ligament injury (475). This kind of problem can't be treated properly at home and requires prompt medical attention.

**472.** *How can I tell if my dog has a broken leg?* The dog will be in extreme pain; she'll hold the leg up, and she won't be able to put any weight on it. The leg will become very swollen in a very short time; it may also be limp, swinging loose or hanging at an odd angle. If you can get the dog to a vet quickly, just pick her up carefully and try to avoid bumping the damaged limb or putting pressure on it (452). When no vet is available right away, you should wrap the leg in a soft bandage (474). In the case of a simple fracture, the purpose of the bandage is just to insulate the limb and keep it somewhat immobile, but for a compound fracture (a break in which the bone is sticking through the surface of the skin) the bandage is important protection from contamination. If you find a compound fracture, wash the wound off with water as thoroughly as you can, bandage the leg, and keep it bandaged until you get the dog to your vet. Go quickly, because this is one of the most serious kinds of breaks.

*473. What are the signs of other types of broken bones?*   The most serious kind of broken bone is a back or neck injury. If the dog is completely immobilized or unable to stand and obviously in a great deal of pain, he could be suffering from a broken back or neck. It's important that you minimize the stress to the injured area as you take the dog to your vet. Undue movement or pressure could aggravate the condition and turn a temporary injury into permanent paralysis. Carry the dog on a makeshift stretcher—a blanket or a flat piece of wood will do. Other types of broken bones are usually not this critical and may be much less obvious. Broken ribs will be very hard to spot without an x-ray, unless they're very severely damaged; the dog may have a chronic pain around her chest. A dog with a broken pelvis will be unable to walk without great difficulty, and a dog with a broken jaw will have a lot of trouble eating and the animal's teeth will be out of alignment. A broken jaw will also make the dog's face swell up.

*474. Should I try to put a splint around a broken bone?*   No. A splint is hard to apply properly, and it may do more harm than good. The best way to insulate a broken limb is to wrap it in a bandage of thick cotton and gauze, padding it as much as possible, and then taping it together. If these materials aren't available, you can improvise using old clothes or towels. Just pad the break as much as possible and take the animal to your vet to have the leg set.

*475. If there are no broken bones, what could cause a dog to hold his hind leg up and refuse to put any weight on it at all?*   If the dog was in an accident, or the condition came on suddenly in the middle of some rough activity that involved a lot of jumping and twisting, it's probably a cruciate ligament injury, essentially the same kind of knee damage that plagues football quarterbacks. Very simply, a ligament in the knee breaks. When this happens, the dog will hold the leg up high to protect it, and the knee will be very lax. In 75 to 80 percent of these cases, surgery is required to repair the damage: the operation can be performed by any good vet. In some instances, the leg may heal without surgery, because the ligament has been stretched instead of snapped. Only a careful veterinary exam can detect which condition is present.

*476. We had a fire, and our dog was caught in the house with a lot of smoke. Is this dangerous? He seems all right now.*   Smoke inhalation is rarely a problem for dogs because they're so low to the ground. Nevertheless, even if the dog seems all right, take him to your vet anyway. At first, there may only be a minor sign of trouble—a dry, raspy cough that doesn't seem serious. But thermal and chemical burns from caustic smoke can damage lung tissue and devitalize it, leaving the dog vulnerable to bacterial and viral infections that in turn can lead to pneumonia (639). The dry cough can begin to produce mucus and even blood in a day or two. Also watch the dog for shallow, rapid breathing and lethargy. These are all signs of smoke-damaged lungs that will need medical attention.

*477. How do you treat a dog that's been badly burned?*   This requires medical attention. In the meantime, keep the wound clean and moist—wrap it with a wet towel. Above all, waste no time in getting the animal to a vet. A dog can lose a lot of fluid through a burn and the animal can become dehydrated. This can lead to kidney failure.

*478. How should I treat milder burns, like a foot pad that's been burned from stepping on a lit cigarette?* This is something that can be taken care of at home. Run cold water over the burn for 10 or 15 minutes, then apply petroleum jelly and cover it with a bandage. Make sure the bandage is well padded and soft where it touches the skin, particularly in the case of a burned foot pad. Change the bandage every third day, and make sure the circulation isn't cut off if the bandage is applied to an extremity. (The leg will start to swell above the bandage if it's put on too tightly.) It takes a burned pad about a month to fully heal. The dog's callus will come 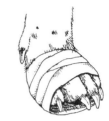 off, so you'll have to be careful about where he walks, even after the bandage is removed. Check the paw every day to make sure that nothing has become imbedded in the tender, exposed flesh.

*479. What kind of first aid is needed if my dog has been burned by a caustic chemical?* Flush the burn thoroughly with water. In the case of stove cleaners and other acidic cleaning fluids, put sodium bicarbonate (baking soda) on the skin to neutralize the acid. If the acid has been *swallowed*, feed the dog egg whites to neutralize the acid and go to the vet *right away* for more extensive help (488).

*480. What are the signs that a dog has gotten an electric shock from chewing an electrical wire?* Look for burn marks on the dog's tongue and lips; they may be swollen and discolored a bluish black. The pupils of the dog's eyes may be dilated, and he could seem stunned. In extreme cases, the shock will cause the dog's heart to stop and the animal will be unable to breathe. You'll have to administer mouth-to-mouth resuscitation and heart massage immediately (446, 448). This type of burn to a dog's mouth can have serious results. It can damage the animal's tongue so badly that portions of it will have to be removed; the shock can also result in pulmonary edema—fluid in the lungs—which must be treated medically.

*481. What should I do for a dog that's been rescued from near drowning?* Pound lightly and rhythmically on the dog's chest with both hands to help him cough up water from the lungs. Twenty or 30 times a minute should be about right. In an extreme situation, apply mouth-to-mouth resuscitation (446). The *kind* of water the dog was swimming in makes a big difference as far as the animal's chances of survival go. Salt water is very nearly equal in osmotic pressure to the dog's blood, so it draws blood into the dog's lungs. When this happens, the dog can drown in his own bodily fluids. Fresh water doesn't have this same drawing capacity, so there's more time to act and less fluid to be expelled.

*482. My dog has something in his eye. How should I get it out?* If it's loose, try to flush it out with an eyewash. You could also just gently pour warm water or a boric acid solution over the eye. If something's stuck in the eyeball, *don't* try to pull it out; this could make the eye collapse. Liberal flushing with water will help combat infection, but don't waste too much time on this. Just get to your veterinarian as quickly as you can—this is a serious condition that needs fast attention.

*483. My dog's eye has slipped out of its socket. What should I do?* This happens frequently when little breeds of "pop-eyed" dogs, such as pugs and Pekinese, get into a fight. It's important to keep the eye moist—drape a wet cloth pad over the eye and make sure it stays damp. The dog should be kept as still as possible and be taken to your vet immediately.

**484. Should I try to take porcupine quills out of my dog's face and paws?**  This is *very* painful to the dog, so you should only do it in an *absolute* emergency, when you can't get to your veterinarian for some time. With a pair of pliers, grip the quill up where it meets the dog's flesh; then just yank it out. Make sure you get it all. A porcupine's quill is designed to burrow deeper and deeper, and it can cause a lot of anguish and damage if it breaks and some of it remains in the dog's flesh. That's why you should have the dog checked out by your vet as soon as you can to make sure the quills are all out and no infection has developed. If you can get to a vet without too much trouble, it's best to let the doctor take care of the whole operation; that way, the animal can be anesthetized before the quills are removed.

**485. How do you remove a fishhook from a dog's mouth?**  In an emergency, you can take the hook out yourself—but you'll probably need to have help holding the dog still and keeping his mouth open (463). First aid in such a situation requires some deft fingers and a pair of wire cutters. A hook can't just be pulled back out because one end is barbed and the other has a round loop where the line is attached; one of these has to be cut off in order for you to pull the hook out without ripping the dog's flesh. If the barb is under the surface of the skin, carefully push it on through until it's exposed. Then either clip it off and take the wire out backwards or cut off the loop and pull the wire out by the barbed end. However, it's very doubtful that a dog will sit still for any of this. The safest and easiest thing to do is to take the dog to your vet so the hook can be extracted while the dog is anesthetized. Even if you get the hook out by yourself, and the dog should still be examined by your vet.

**486. Will it be all right in an emergency to give my dog some old antibiotics I have left over from my last case of the flu?**  For something minor—such as a cut, a dog or cat bite, or an external wound that's obviously infected—it's permissible to give the dog one of the common antibiotics—*but only until it's possible to check with a vet and get a prescription.* For drugs like ampicillin or tetracycline, the dose for a 25-pound dog should be 250 milligrams three times a day. Make sure this interim treatment is consistent. It does no good to give the dog one or two pills and then stop. In order to be effective, they must be administered regularly for at least five days. During that time, it should be possible to get professional advice. WARNING: This treatment is permissible *only* in the case of an *obvious external wound*. Don't give your pet antibiotics if you think he has a cold. It could be a virus, and the antibiotics could make it worse.

**487. Should I worry if my dog accidentally swallows illegal drugs such as marijuana or LSD?**  Something as powerful as LSD can obviously leave a dog disoriented. It's possible that the experience could change his personality for quite a long time afterward, if not permanently. On the other hand, when dogs consume hashish or marijuana in any sizeable quantity it usually just puts them to sleep. If a dog is under the influence of any disorienting drug, try to keep the surroundings as familiar and reassuring as possible, and be cautious in handling the animal. If the dog is unconscious, or has consumed a large amount of a drug, take him to your vet.

**488. What poisons do dogs encounter the most, and what can be done when a dog is poisoned?** It's very rare for a dog to be poisoned at all, but here are some of the most common poisons: *Ethylene glycol:* This sweet tasting, toxic chemical is the main ingredient in automobile antifreeze. If you see a dog drinking it, don't wait for signs of poisoning to appear. Rush the animal to a vet and give the dog ethyl alcohol (any alcoholic beverage, even beer) as an antidote while you're in transit. The symptoms of antifreeze poisoning are excessive salivation, vomiting, convulsions, and delirium. *Rat poison:* There are several kinds of rat poison, and you should try to find out what kind your dog has eaten. Induce vomiting by giving the dog about a tablespoon of hydrogen peroxide for each 10 pounds of the dog's weight. Or give the dog a spoonful of table salt at the back of the mouth. Then rush the dog to your vet. There may be no symptoms of rat poisoning if the dog hasn't eaten a large amount, and this type of poison isn't usually fatal unless the dog has eaten a great deal, up to half his body weight. Advanced poisoning will cause internal hemorrhaging. *Bleach:* Do *not* induce vomiting. Just hurry to the animal hospital. If no other help is available, give the dog mustard or egg whites to decrease the bleach's absorption into the system. *Gasoline, kerosene, drain cleaners:* Do *not* induce vomiting. Rush to the vet. *Lead-based paints:* Dogs occasionally swallow lead-based paints if they chew on old woodwork. (Newer paints don't contain lead.) This form of poisoning will cause extreme abdominal pains and convulsions. There's a specific antidote for lead poisoning, and any well-equipped animal hospital should have it on hand. *Arsenic:* Arsenic is another poison for which there is a specific antidote. Symptoms of this type of exposure will be excessive vomiting and abdominal pain. Give the dog some baking soda and rush him to the vet. *Organophosphate pesticides:* This type of poisoning may come from eating the poison or by exposure to agricultural spraying. If the dog has the pesticide on his skin, wash him thoroughly with an alkaline detergent and consult your vet. For poison that's been swallowed, induce vomiting. If the dog is already showing convulsions and other erratic behavior, there may have been neurological damage. Take the dog to the vet as quickly as possible. *Strychnine:* Seizures and convulsions are also associated with this type of poisoning. The dog may react strangely to noises, and seem to be suffering from hallucinations. Strychnine can cause paralysis and kidney damage. The best treatment is to induce vomiting, then see your vet.

**489. Aren't there plants that can poison a dog?** Yes, although this type of poisoning is very unusual. In most cases, the dog will just be very sick to his stomach. But even though they're rarely fatal, plant poisoning *can* be dangerous to the dog's health. The most common plant poisonings occur with poinsettias, philodendrons, and Dieffenbachia. After the animal chews on the plant, he'll begin to salivate a great deal. Then he'll suffer from paralysis of the tongue, his mucus membranes will be irritated, and he'll have difficulty swallowing and breathing. A general debilitation and listlessness will follow. If the dog is severely ill, take him to your vet. Otherwise, the condition will usually pass on its own.

**490. Is there a universal antidote for poisoning in dogs like the one we learned for people?** The volume and variety of toxic chemicals in the world today have made such a simple formula obsolete, for people as well as dogs. Your first aid procedures should depend on what the dog has swallowed (488). The main thing to do is to get the dog to a vet as quickly as possible. If you can't get to a vet, you can also try calling the local poison-control center. Whatever antidote is given to a human being will also apply to your dog.

**491. How should I treat bee stings and other insect bites?**   Bee stings and insect bites usually go unnoticed; dogs don't often find them as painful as we do. They may just suffer from a little swelling around the bite, and sometimes they break out in hives. The symptoms usually go away in a few hours. To make the dog a little more comfortable, give her some aspirin (308) and then watch to make sure that the situation doesn't get worse. If the swelling isn't gone in a day or the animal begins to have trouble breathing, take her to the vet for further treatment.

**492. What should I do if my dog is bitten by a snake?**   A snakebite wound will cause a large swelling, usually on the face or front limbs, and the dog will be in great pain. A *poisonous* snakebite requires emergency medical help as fast as possible. While you're on your way to the vet, keep the dog still so that the venom circulates as little as possible (you may have to exert a lot of force to do this). If the bite is on the dog's leg, apply a tourniquet tightly, but not so tight that it completely closes off the circulation (466). Do not allow anyone other than a vet to remove the tourniquet or loosen it unless it's been on for a minimum of two hours. Treat the bite itself by making a cut over each fang wound and sucking out as much of the venom as you can. If possible, use suction cups like the ones provided in a snake-bite kit. If a veterinarian is nearby, the suction treatment isn't so important—getting the dog to the animal hospital should be your primary concern.

**493. My dog acts like there's something stuck in her ear. Should I try to remove it?**   Examine the ear, using a flashlight. If you can see the object, try to get a grip on it with tweezers, then lubricate the ear with mineral oil and gently pull the object out. If it seems stuck, don't try to force it out; take the animal to the vet. You should also take the dog to the vet if she's shaking her head violently and you can't see anything in the ear.

**494. How do you recognize frostbite, and how is it treated in a dog?**   Frostbite is very much like a burn. It usually affects the foot pads. Initially, there's a numbness to the feet, as well as frozen flesh. Then the affected limb will begin to swell and become very sore. What's happened, in effect, is that a portion of the dog's foot has been killed by the cold. The pad will become grayish colored, and layers of skin and fur will begin to slough off. If left untreated, gangrene will usually set in, and the dog could quickly die of blood poisoning. If you find a dog that's been exposed to severe cold and the animal limps and seems in pain when he walks, have him examined by a vet as soon as possible.

## Common Ailments: Vomiting, Diarrhea, Constipation

**495. What could be wrong if my dog starts vomiting?**   Several things can be wrong, but no matter what the problem is, if the dog continues to vomit for longer than 48 hours, take him to your vet. Prolonged vomiting can make the animal become dehydrated (293). It's especially important not to let this go untreated in puppies because they can lose a lot of vitamins and nutrients at a crucial time in their lives, and the danger of dehydration is even greater for them than it is for older dogs.

The most common and obvious reason for vomiting is an upset stomach. This is a particular problem for a "garbage hound," a dog that eats whatever is around. If your dog has an upset stomach, withhold food for 12 hours and give him small amounts of water or ice cubes to lick (too much water at one time isn't likely to stay down). Also give the dog some kind of human antacid to settle his stomach (a child's dose for a small dog, an adult dose for a dog that weighs over 10 lbs., and in severe cases a double dose for dogs over 60 lbs.). Vomiting can also be a sign that the dog has internal parasites. Puppies will sometimes vomit up worms, along with food and mucus (31,32). If adult dogs have whipworms, they may vomit in the morning when they don't have anything in their stomachs and are feeling nauseous from the worm infestation in their intestines (594). A third possible cause of vomiting is an intestinal virus. This will usually be followed by diarrhea, and generally it just runs its course. Take care that the dog doesn't become dehydrated while he rides out the illness, and check with your vet if it goes on more than two days.

**496. What can cause a dog to have chronic diarrhea?**   If the diarrhea is intermittent and seems to come back every week or two, have your dog checked for worms. If there's no sign of worms and your dog is the nervous type, the problem may be stress. It could also be colitis, an inflamed colon. Most vets can provide you with a commercial diet for colitis that will ease the problem. You can also experiment with a diet of a little canned food, some all-bran, rice, and eggs. This may be helpful if the dog doesn't like the commercial colitis remedy. If the diet alone doesn't reduce the inflammation, try the diet and the medicine in combination. You can work out the proportions with your vet. If the dog seems very weak and feverish, and has profound and bloody diarrhea, the animal could be suffering from a bacterial disease known as salmonellosis. This is highly contagious and it can also be transmitted to human beings. Salmonellosis must be diagnosed through a fecal culture test, and once it's discovered it should be treated with antiobiotics immediately.

**497. My dog has been drinking a lot more water lately and passing a greater amount of urine than he used to. What could be wrong?**   Higher water consumption and a significant increase in the amount of urine are symptoms of three possible disorders —kidney disease, Cushing's disease, or diabetes. *Kidney disease* causes a breakdown in the kidney's ability to cleanse the blood; it can be a result of aging or of a toxic reaction to poisoning. Kidney damage can't be reversed, but the dog's health *can* be improved with changes in his diet to reduce the amount of protein that's taken in (180,637). In the latter stages of kidney failure, the dog will become nauseous and stop eating, a response that also comes with Cushing's disease and diabetes. *Cushing's disease* is a metabolic disorder that affects human beings as well as dogs. It occurs when the body produces too much steroid, a hormone manufactured by the adrenal glands. Steroids are used by doctors as an anti-inflammatory treatment for ailing joints; they're naturally produced when a person becomes excited, and make your heart race. Too much of the steroid hormone will cause a dog to drink more water; urinate more; have a thin, sparce coat and flaky skin; and become nauseous and potbellied. It's possible for a dog to contract Cushing's disease as a side-effect of some *other* treatment, as steroids are one of the most commonly prescribed drugs for dogs; they're used to combat arthritis, allergy, and unspecified dermatitis, and even in cancer therapy. *Diabetes* is a disease that can only be controlled rather than cured. Like its human counterpart, canine diabetes involves the production of insufficient amounts of insulin. Signs of the disease include excessive water intake and urination, a voracious appetite, obesity, and a sweet-scented breath. Our ability to control diabetes depends on how soon it's detected, so take your dog in for a check-up if you see any of these symptoms. Once the condition is diagnosed, expect to make some changes in the dog's diet.

**498. My dog has diarrhea and has been vomiting a little bit. Is this serious, or can I treat it at home?**   If there are other symptoms present—if the dog is lethargic, has a high temperature, and is vomiting excessively (six or seven times a day for a couple of days), or if you see blood in the vomit or diarrhea—consult your vet. These could be symptoms of a condition that requires medical attention. If the dog is just having ordinary diarrhea, and even vomiting a little bit, he's probably suffering from a reaction to eating spoiled food or garbage or, at the worst, an internal parasite. If he hasn't been checked for worms recently, you should take a stool sample to the vet. Meanwhile, don't feed the dog for 24 hours. Give him only small amounts of water (or put ice cubes in his water dish) and give him any of the over-the-counter anti-diarrheal preparations. Give small dogs a child's dose, and an adult portion to dogs over forty pounds. After 24 hours, feed the dog small meals by dividing a normal day's food into three or four servings. This can be supplemented with chicken or beef broth, and boiled meat and rice can be substituted for part of the canned food the dog normally eats. Cottage cheese and chicken are also good substitutes for regular dog food. Continue this diet for two or three days, and if the dog doesn't improve, consult your vet.

**499. What's wrong with a dog that strains to urinate and produces nothing, or very little?**   This could be a bladder infection, bladder stones, or possibly a prostate problem. A *bladder infection* can be helped with a treatment of vitamin C and antibiotics. The vitamin C acidifies the urine, which in turn reduces the growth of bacteria and promotes healing. Simple bladder infections are more a problem for female dogs because a male dog's bladder isn't as accessible to contamination. *Bladder stones* can affect either sex, and they may become a severe problem. If the dog is unable to urinate or dribbles a little bloody urine or just blood, the bladder is probably blocked with stones. These are caused by chronic bladder infections or genetic metabolic problems. A female dog may pass the stones out, but only the smallest ones can pass out of a male dog. If a male dog lifts his leg and tries repeatedly to urinate and nothing comes out, or if only a few drops of blood appear, he needs immediate attention. The bladder has to be emptied, and the stones must be removed surgically. If your dog has had incidences of bladder stones, take him off dry food and don't add bone meal to his food. You should also consult with your vet about other diet changes.

**500. My dog strains when he defecates. What could be the problem?**   The dog could have an inflamed prostate gland or a perineal hernia—or he could just be constipated. If the dog is having trouble defecating *and* urinating, if he seems to have an unspecified pain around his hind end, and if there's a small amount of greenish or yellowish discharge from his penis, his prostate gland could be infected. In mild cases, this can be treated with antibiotics and estrogen compounds; more severe problems require surgery. If there's a bulge on either side of the dog's anus while he's defecating, the animal could be suffering from a perineal hernia. This usually occurs in older dogs, seven years and up, and it requires surgery or medical treatment. If you suspect your dog has a perineal hernia take the animal to your vet for help. The third major possibility, and the mildest, is simple constipation—when a dog goes for two or more days without a bowel movement. As a laxative, add vegetable oil to the dog's food (one teaspoon for every 10 pounds of the dog's weight) or just put some petroleum jelly on the dog's upper lip. When the jelly is licked off, it's swallowed and it lubricates the dog's digestive tract. You could also buy a stool softener at the pharmacy. Ask your vet about the proper dosage.

## Eye, Ear, and Mouth Problems

**501. My dog's eyes are watery and they seem to be constantly draining. What's wrong?** Excessive tearing is usually harmless, just a sign that the tear ducts are clogged. Tears that would normally be going through a channel in the dog's nose to the throat are now coming out the eyes. Our own tear system works much the same way, draining out the eyes and down the throat. Poodles are particularly troubled by faulty tear ducts. They're often born without the complete tear apparatus, or with a defective one, and they suffer from a continual drainage down the face. It's a natural thing, and not a disease or a dangerous disorder. However, in especially bad cases the dog's tear ducts may need to be surgically cleaned. Excessive tearing can become a problem when the dog's face is continuously wet and the eyes become inflamed from having moist hair around them constantly. This creates a potential breeding ground for infection, and you should consult your vet on how to deal with it.

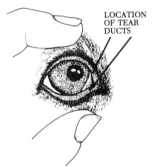

LOCATION OF TEAR DUCTS

**502. My dog has a large, pink knot in the corner of his eye. What is it?** This condition, which usually affects pups of the short-nosed breeds, is known as cherry eye. It

PINK KNOT

*Cherry eye*

appears when a tear gland connected to the third eyelid (the nictitating membrane) becomes inflamed. This gland is a minor, auxilliary supplier of lubricant to the eye. Because it's located in a vulnerable place, it's more prone to infection than the other tear glands further inside the dog's head. Cherry eye can be treated with corticosteroids, but the gland may have to be surgically removed, along with the nictitating membrane, if there's no improvement through the drug treatment.

**503. What's making my dog's eyes red? They're giving off a mucus discharge too.** This is probably simple conjunctivitis, also known as "pink eye," an infection of the conjunctiva, the membrane that lines the lids and part of the eye. It isn't usually serious, and it can be cleared up by wiping away the yellow-green mucus three times a day and washing out the eye with a boric acid wash, which is available over the counter at drugstores. An average case of conjunctivitis should clear up in about three days. If there's no improvement in two days, or if the infection gets worse at any time, the dog needs to go to the vet. If there's anything at all wrong with the eye itself—an ulcer on the clear surface of the cornea or cloudiness developing within the eye—have the dog examined by your vet.

*504. My dog's eyes always seem to be red. Does that mean they're infected?* Some dogs have eyelids that naturally turn out or in a little bit, and this causes them to have a chronic, low-grade form of conjunctivitis all the time because these lid formations are a constant irritation to the eye. Corrective surgery is possible if the eye is actually being damaged; otherwise, the problem isn't significant. Basset hounds and St. Bernards are the two breeds that most often have lids that turn out. Irish setters, golden retrievers, and bulldogs often have lids that roll inward.

*505. Do dogs suffer from glaucoma?* Glaucoma is an increase in pressure within the eye. It shows up occasionally in dogs, and when it does it comes on rapidly. The signs of glaucoma are a bulging of the eye, continued dilation of the pupil, redness in the white of the eye, constant tearing, cloudiness of the eye, and impaired vision. Glaucoma is usually treated with drugs, but surgery is sometimes performed.

*506. Our dog has a cataract in one eye, but she gets along all right. Can this cause any other problems we should be aware of?* If the dog can see well enough to live normally, I wouldn't worry about it, particularly if she's an old dog whose ability to withstand surgery might be limited. However, there *is* one potential problem; cataracts can lead to glaucoma (505, 631, 632).

*507. My dog's ear is swelling up. Why?* Excessive head shaking, perhaps from ear mites (566) or another irritation, can sometimes rupture a blood vessel in the dog's ear. The swelling can be minor, or the ear can be *really* distended. This problem usually happens to hounds with very floppy ears, and the only cure is to have your vet surgically drain the ear. Don't try to drain the ear at home.

*508. What do you recommend to keep flies from biting my dog's ears?* A dog's ears are very vulnerable, and since they're a favorite place for flies to bite, this can cause a bad infection. If the ear is sore and badly bitten, it can be treated with antibiotic ointment, but have your vet look at the ear if it doesn't show signs of healing in two days. To keep the flies from further damaging and harassing the dog, use one of the common over-the-counter insect repellents.

*509. My dog has had ear infections off and on for some time. Could this affect her hearing?* Yes. Chronic, repetitive ear infections can cause the tissues around the ear canal to become so inflamed and swollen that the canal is almost completely closed up. This doesn't allow for any drainage, so the animal's ability to hear is reduced. This condition can be corrected surgically by cutting down the side of the canal and enlarging it to insure proper drainage.

*510. What causes deafness in dogs?* Most of the time, this is simply caused by aging; over the years, there's a degeneration of the auditory nerve. Sometimes it's hard to tell whether a dog is becoming deaf or is just mentally and physically slow to respond. All these conditions come on with senility. In younger dogs, deafness can be a genetic problem, or it can be the result of recurrent ear infections.

*511. What could make a dog's gums turn bright red?* Red gums and very bad breath could be signs of trench mouth, a gum infection which can be treated with antibiotics. Another possibility is periodontal disease; in this case, the teeth will have bad plaque stains (141). There are other problems that can change the appearance of a dog's mouth, and obviously this kind of a symptom shouldn't be ignored.

**512. *I think my dog is growing an upper fang. Is this possible?*** Yes. This happens a lot with smaller dogs. The baby teeth don't always fall out, and the adult teeth start growing beside them. If you see an extra fang in your dog's mouth, take the animal to your vet to have the baby tooth pulled.

**513. *Does an excessive overbite or underbite present any danger to my dog's health?*** Unless it's a very extreme case, there's no reason to worry. The upper jaw may be longer or shorter than the lower one, but this doesn't have any significance unless you've bred the dog for show—in that case, the dog simply wouldn't be a successful show dog.

**514. *Do dogs suffer from tonsilitis?*** Tonsilitis can occur in every breed, but the smaller breeds are more prone to it. If a dog *is* prone to tonsilitis it usually comes on when the animal is about 3 to 6 months old. If your dog has reached this age without suffering from tonsilitis, he's unlikely to ever have it. The symptoms are constant gagging and difficulty swallowing. The condition can be treated with drugs, providing it isn't too severe. In chronic cases, the tonsils may have to be removed.

**515. *My dog's face is swollen under the right eye, her mouth seems to be hurting, and her appetite is off. Is this a tooth problem?*** It sounds like an abscessed tooth. This usually occurs with the carnasal tooth, the largest molar in the dog's mouth, located in the rear of the upper jaw (256). This condition will also cause a dog's breath to become foul-smelling. Occasionally the abscess can break open, leaving a small hole in the dog's face under the eye. This will remain a chronic problem until the tooth is pulled.

**516. *My dog seems to be drooling a lot. What could be wrong?*** Excessive drooling could be a sign that your dog has an abscessed tooth or a gum infection (both of which will also be accompanied by bad breath), or it could be caused by an inflamed salivary gland. Of course, St. Bernards and some other breeds drool quite a bit anyway, because of the way their lips are formed. The sign you should watch for is drooling that's abnormal for *your* dog.

## Respiratory Ailments

**517. *Can dogs catch colds and flu from people?*** Generally no. Most viruses can't be transmitted between human beings and dogs.

**518. *Why is my dog sneezing?*** Your dog could have inhaled dust—or he could be suffering from a mild upper-respiratory virus or sinus infection. This is nothing to worry about, and it will usually pass on its own. If it continues and you see a discharge, your dog may have a stubborn sinus infection, and this will require some medical attention. For milder conditions, aspirin will help (308). Sneezing could also result when the dog has a small obstruction lodged in his nasal passage; this sometimes happens with seed pods. If the sneezing is especially violent and persistent, the dog could need help in getting the obstruction removed. Look the dog over, and if you can't see the object protruding—and especially if there's blood coming from the dog's nose—go to your vet for help. There are two other conditions that may cause a dog to sneeze—a tumor in the nose (marked by sneezing and nosebleeds) and periodontal disease, which sometimes affects the dog's sinuses and makes him sneeze (141).

**519. My dog makes snorts that sound almost like sneezing, and this goes on for several minutes without stopping. What's wrong?** Dogs have a habit called reverse sneezing; it's a kind of snorting attack during which they inhale very rapidly. It usually lasts for about 10 minutes, and it may come on about once or twice a week. Reverse sneezing may be caused by postnasal drip, although this isn't the only possible reason. In any case, there's no need to worry; the animal is in no danger. This is just a way of clearing the nasal passages and throat.

**520. My dog is coughing a lot. What could be wrong with him?** If the dog was recently boarded in a kennel and has developed a rasping, strong cough, I would suspect that he has tracheobronchitis (523). If the dog is less than seven years old, asthma (522) and distemper (608) are also possibilities. Pneumonia (639) could also cause coughing, but there would be other noticeable symptoms. Coughing could also indicate the presence of parasitic heartworms (583) or it may be caused by genetic defects. In an older dog, one that's 10 years old or more, coughing at night may be a sign of heart problems (619).

**521. Our poodle has trouble sometimes when we go for a walk. He coughs and seems to be gagging. Could the collar be choking him?** It's very likely that your poodle has a collapsing trachea, a genetic problem peculiar to poodles and some other small breeds. The weakened structure of the dog's trachea allows it to collapse, usually when the dog becomes excited or when pressure is placed on his throat. When this happens, the dog goes into a fit of coughing that sounds much more serious than it really is—this harsh, honking cough forces the trachea open again. This problem is only dangerous in very severe cases.

**522. What affects asthma in dogs, and how can it be controlled?** Asthmatic coughing seems to grow worse in most dogs when they become excited; in extremes of humidity, heat, cold, and dryness; and after they drink water (which puts pressure on the chest and the upper air passages). Asthma isn't a life-threatening condition, so you should just concentrate on keeping the animal comfortable. Your vet can prescribe medications, and aspirin sometimes helps too (308).

**523. My dog was coughing so hard that I thought he was choking on something, but there's nothing stuck in his throat and he isn't bringing up any phlegm. What could be wrong?** This sounds like tracheobronchitis, or kennel cough, an upper respiratory disease that's highly contagious and spreads as fast as the flu. It's marked by a deep, unproductive cough that's similar to whooping cough in children. Kennel cough isn't very serious, but it sounds terrible, and it *can* lead to pneumonia if it goes untreated. You can treat this problem at home for the most part, using over-the-counter human cough suppressants and expectorants. You should also contact your vet about the possibility of using antibiotics to guard against further infection. The disease will usually clear up in about 10 days, and if it doesn't you should take the dog in to your vet. If you notice any *other* symptoms developing—such as mucus from the nostrils, lethargy, or fever—or if there's any worsening of the problem, go to your vet immediately.

**524. *Isn't there a vaccine that can prevent kennel cough?*** Yes. It's part of the combination shot that goes along with the dog's annual distemper vaccination (281), and it's about 75 percent effective. Kennel cough caused by a multitude of viruses, and some of these may be somewhat resistant to the vaccine. However, even if your dog *does* come down with kennel cough after being vaccinated, he's likely to have a much less severe case.

**525. *Is it possible that my dog is coughing because he's allergic to something?*** This is unlikely. Dogs usually show an allergic reaction by developing a rash (527).

## Skin Conditions, Sores, Abscesses

**526. *Do dogs get sunburned?*** No. Their coats protect them from the sun's rays. However, dogs with unpigmented noses *can* suffer from a condition called "collie nose syndrome." This is very much like sun poisoning in human beings; it causes a kind of ulcerous sore—the dog's nose becomes red, puffy, and sore. Have this checked by your vet because it's possible that it can lead to skin cancer. "Collie nose" can be prevented by using suntan lotion or some other protective substance.

**527. *What are the signs that a dog has an allergy?*** Dogs are allergic to most of the same things that bother people—pollen, feathers, dust, molds, and so forth (529). If your dog has an allergy, it will usually show up when the animal is about 2 to 4 years old. And it's liable to happen in the summer and early fall because these are the biggest allergy seasons for dogs. The first signs will be mild scratching; this intensifies to severe itching, which in turn can lead to open sores on the skin from constant irritation. (In the case of a flea-bite allergy, the worst signs will show up near the lower back and tail.) Other general signs of allergies are licking at the paws and rubbing the eyes. On the other hand, sneezing is more often a sign of sinus problems or of something that's caught in the dog's nose (518).

**528. *How do you find out what specific thing a dog is allergic to? How is the allergy treated?*** Just as with people, dog allergies are diagnosed through the often tedious trial-and-error process of a skin test. Once an allergen is isolated, the easiest way to stop the allergy is to simply remove the allergen from the dog's environment. If this can't be done, then two kinds of treatment are possible. The dog can be given steroids to eliminate the symptoms of the allergy or the dog can be gradually desensitized by receiving weekly doses of the allergen and developing an immunity to it. The second option has some important advantages because a dog shouldn't be kept on steroids for more than 3 or 4 weeks at a time. However, without the steroids the allergy returns, and allergies have a way of becoming worse as time goes by. If a dog starts having allergy problems when she's young, or if she's particularly susceptible to an allergy, then hyposensitization is a good choice. Unfortunately, the treatment takes 1 to 2 years to carry out, and it can be expensive.

**529. What causes a dog to break out in hives, and what should I do about it?**   Insect bites and other irritations cause this allergic reaction. In severe cases, the dog may need corticosteroids, but most of the time the condition will clear up in a day or two. Give the dog aspirin to make him more comfortable (308).

**530. My dog has body odor, flaking skin, and little sores on his back. What's wrong?** This is probably seborrhea, a problem that arises from abnormal oil production in the dog's skin. It's incurable, but it *can* be controlled. Start by cleaning the dog with a medicated shampoo; follow the shampoo with a bath-oil rinse (116). If the sore spots are mild, you can just treat them with antibiotic ointment or powder. If they're more severe they should be cared for by your vet.

**531. What could it mean if my dog has a swollen lymph node?**   The body's lymphatic system fights infection, makes white blood cells, and filters the blood, so a swollen lymph node probably is caused by a minor infection in the area. For example, if a dog gets an infected paw, the node under that leg usually enlarges. A lymph node

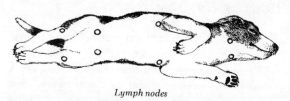

*Lymph nodes*

can also become abscessed and swell up when there's no other source of infection in the area, or it can enlarge because of lymphosarcoma, a form of leukemia (630). If the dog has a lymph node that's consistently swollen, and there's no obvious cause, or if more than one node swells up at the same time, then it's a good idea to have a small part of the affected node removed for a biopsy and examined for signs of cancer. If the node is swollen for two or three weeks with no visible sign of infection, a biopsy should be done as quickly as possible. If the dog *does* have cancer, her chances for survival are greater when the disease is detected *early*.

**532. What can be wrong with a dog's paw that would make her lick and chew at it continuously?**   The first possibility is an allergy (527). The second is simply boredom. Dogs groom and lick and fuss over their feet when there's nothing to bark at and nothing to sniff or chase. If the dog's paw seems red, this may just be a result of constant licking—a dog's saliva has enzymes in it that tend to leave a reddish stain on the animal's fur when she licks a spot repeatedly. Just to be sure, though, you should examine the paw for signs of punctures or cuts. If the paw is swollen and you see a hole or a cut, this could be caused by a foreign object, such as a thorn or a piece of glass, that the dog has been unable to remove. It's likely that anything you could get out with tweezers, the dog would have already removed with her teeth, but if you *do* see the object, remove it and swab the paw with a mild antiseptic. Repeat this cleaning twice a day until the sore spot clears up. If the object isn't visible any longer, but there does seem to have been a puncture, the object may have to be extracted through minor surgery, and the dog will require antibiotics to prevent infection. This is a matter for your vet to handle.

**533. My dog has been licking the same place on his stomach over and over again until it's started to look really red and sore. What's wrong with him?**   Human beings usually know better than to scratch any itchy place too much because this only makes it worse. But dogs just know that the place itches, so they scratch or lick or chew at it, trying to get some relief. This turns a little itch into an inflamed, potentially infected area known as a "hot spot." If you catch a hot spot early, you can clip off the hair around it, wash it well with soap and water about three times a day, and treat it with antibiotic powder or ointment. Keep up this treatment for about 5 days and the hot spot should clear up. If it gets worse and starts to look infected, take the dog to the vet. If your dog just won't leave the spot alone, you can make an "Elizabethan collar" for him (313).

**534. *A large, soft bump that looks like a sore has formed on my dog's skin. What is this?*** The sudden appearance of a soft, red, hairless bump on a dog's skin, especially around the anus, is an abscess. If the bump hasn't opened, put warm compresses on it every 2 hours for 10 minutes at a time. This will make the abscess burst and release the pus and bacterial debris that's been building up. Once it opens, clean it with water, then hydrogen peroxide, keeping it open for about four days so that it has a good opportunity to flush out. This antiseptic cleansing should be continued for about five days, and by then the abscess should be healing well. If not, go to the vet and have it checked. Cat bites and other puncture wounds may cause an abscess, but the most common place for dogs to have abscesses is in the anal scent glands; they develop when the dog doesn't have a proper diet and the contents of the glands don't empty during a bowel movement.

**535. *My dog has been scooting her rear end along the ground as if it itches. Is this a sign of trouble?*** When a dog drags her bottom along the ground and is constantly licking her anus, this is a sign that the anal scent glands aren't functioning properly. These glands usually secrete a scented liquid when the dog defecates, but smaller breeds—and dogs fed a soft diet or table scraps—sometimes develop clogged scent glands. When this happens, the glands can become abscessed. If you see your dog scooting, try adding some dry food or rice to her meals. This will firm up her feces and help get the glands going again. If this doesn't solve the problem, you'll have to express the glands by hand, or ask your vet to do this during a check-up. You can feel the glands on each side of the dog's anus. To squeeze out the fluid, just pinch the flesh on each side in a kind of milking motion. This can be done when the dog is outside being bathed or groomed. However, it's a good idea to consult with your vet before making this a regular part of the dog's grooming because the glands tend to lose strength if they're frequently expressed by hand, and they can lose their ability to secrete the fluid naturally. Some dogs never need this kind of attention, some need it frequently.

DUCT

ANAL GLAND

## Muscle and Bone Problems

**536. *What joints give a dog the most trouble?*** Most often it's the dog's knee that becomes sprained (470). The second and third most common injuries occur with the dog's hips (601, 538) and elbows.

**537. *What would make my dog hesitate to bend down and eat from his dish or climb stairs?*** This is characteristic behavior of a dog with disk problems in his neck. The dog may cry out when his head is moved up and down or from side to side, and he may be reluctant to bend over, holding his head in a stiff, tucked-in position. This sort of problem is caused by a deterioration of the cushioning disks between the vertebrae of the spinal column in the dog's neck. If you suspect your dog has cervical disk disease, give him aspirin for the pain (308) and then take him to your vet.

**538. *Is it true that the hip bone in some small dogs falls apart at the joint?*** Poodles and other small dogs suffer from a condition called femoral head necrosis. The head of the thigh bone (the femur) loses blood circulation and the bone cells die, causing a deterioration of the bone where it joins the hip. The animal then begins to limp and experiences a lot of pain. An x-ray can confirm the diagnosis, and surgery will usually improve the situation.

**539. *What are joint mice?*** Shoulder joint mice are little bits of cartilage that break off the shoulder joint and lodge in between the bones. They cause a lot of pain, especially when the dog's leg is extended out in front. This condition shows up at an early age, usually around 9 months or a little later, and it usually affects the larger breeds. Joint mice can only be diagnosed with an x-ray. The surgery required to remove them is complicated. It should only be done by an orthopedic specialist or an experienced vet.

**540. *Isn't there a congenital knee problem that occurs in many small breeds?*** Normally, the patella (kneecap) is supposed to move up and down, not from side to side, over the thighbone (femur). When it *does*, this condition is called luxating patella, and it usually occurs in small breeds, especially toy poodles. The side-to-side motion can cause arthritis to develop, and unless it's been discovered during a routine examination, the limping that results will often be the first sign that something is wrong. Because luxating patella is a birth defect, this condition usually affects *both* legs. It can be repaired with surgery; the operation has a high success rate, but it would be wise only to have it done by an orthopedic specialist.

**541. *Aren't some dogs born with a crippling elbow problem?*** This condition is called ununited anconeal process. The point of the elbow isn't united with the rest of the ulna bone of the leg, and it slips around, causing the elbow to be very unstable. This shows up early in a dog's life as a limp. It can be repaired surgically by removing a piece of the bone, by pinning the two pieces together, and by other surgical techniques. The condition is primarily seen in the smaller breeds.

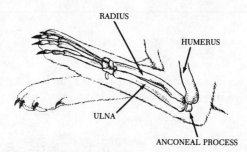

RADIUS

HUMERUS

ULNA

ANCONEAL PROCESS

**542. *My dog has short legs and a long body, and he suffers from occasional back pain. What causes this?*** This kind of pain is common to beagles, basset hounds, and the other short-legged breeds. Their intervertebral disks, which are normally like jelly, tend to calcify prematurely and lose their elasticity. When this happens, any bump or jolt—for example, when the dog jumps up—will cause the disk to move up into the spinal cord, generating a severe shooting pain. The pains won't usually begin to show up until the dog is at least five years old. Surgery can correct the condition.

**543. My dachshund seems to have some back pain, but he isn't incapacitated by it. What can I do for him?** When his back is bothering him, give the dog two baby aspirin three times a day. Be careful, though—you don't want to give the dog *too much* pain-killer, because then he won't be able to *feel* that it's bad to run and jump around, and that will make his back problem worse. Also, it's wise to keep him confined for a few days.

**544. My dog's back pains seem to be getting worse. What can I do?** If you see the dog staggering, or if he seems paralyzed at all, take him to your vet at once. Surgery can help this problem, but the sooner it's done, the better the rate of recovery.

**545. Do dogs suffer from rheumatism?** Yes. Rheumatism (rheumatoid arthritis) is an incurable disease that's related to factors in the blood; it's more severe than the degenerative joint disease that's commonly called arthritis. Rheumatism is diagnosed through a blood test, and its symptoms can be treated with corticosteroids. It's characterized by stiffness of the joints and pain while moving about. The lameness also shifts from day to day, affecting one leg for a while, then moving to another.

**546. Isn't it cruel to amputate a dog's leg?** Certainly not. In the case of bone tumors, severe fractures, and any other situation in which the dog can be saved by removing the limb, it's far and away the best choice. Don't worry that the dog will be crippled. Even very large dogs can get about just fine on three legs.

## External Parasites

**547. Are fleas a serious threat to my dog's health, or just a minor irritation?** Fleas are more than just an annoyance. They're also carriers of tapeworms (576). And dogs can be allergic to flea bites (529). In addition, fleas can drain puppies of so much blood that the pups become anemic.

**548. Won't most fleas come off in a normal bath?** No. Ordinary washing doesn't get rid of fleas. You might eliminate a few by washing them off with the hose or in the rinse water, but mostly you will just wind up with clean fleas.

**549. What's the most effective way of controlling fleas and ticks?** Dipping (550) the dog every 10 days during the warm months of the flea season is the most effective control. This method is thorough, and its killing power is residual. However, in the warmest areas of the South, fleas have become so resistent to pesticides that more frequent dipping or a combination of dipping and flea-protective pills may be necessary. Consult your vet about any extensive use of these methods.

**550. What's the best way to dip a dog?** You can combine a dip with a bath. Be sure not to use flea soap; you don't want to mix pesticides. Before starting, smear petroleum jelly over the dog's eyelids to keep the dip out of his eyes (for male dogs, also cover the animal's scrotum with petroleum jelly—the skin there is very thin and sensitive). Then mix the dip in the prescribed concentration. The dog has to be wet before you dip him, so you should soak him thoroughly before proceeding. If you have a big dog, you can sponge the dip on so that he's well covered. For small dogs, you can put the dip in a plant sprayer. Set the nozzle for a thick spray (a finer mist will get in the dog's eyes) and then just squirt it on. Remember that a dip has to stay on the dog in order to do its work; you can't wipe it off. You *can* damp-dry the dog with a towel to get rid of the excess dip, but let the rest of it dry on his coat. Only dip the dog on days when his coat will dry quickly. Check with the local animal society to see if they offer free dips during the summer.

**551. Is it dangerous for my children to play with the dog after she's been dipped?** Certainly. You don't want the children—or anyone else—to play with the dog while she's still drying after being dipped. In fact, if you have small children, you may not want to use a dip at all because of the residual pesticide left in the animal's coat. An alternative is a weekly bath with a flea shampoo. It isn't as powerful and long-lasting as a dip, but it *is* safer. (555)

**552. Are flea collars bad for a dog's health?** Nearly every method of flea control involves the use of pesticides, but the health risks to the dog are generally minimal, and they're less of a problem than the infections and chronic skin irritations that result from an unchecked flea infestation. There's no solid evidence that flea collars are harmful to dogs, although there *are* some things to be careful about when using them. There are three basic types available—collars that use a skin-absorption method, powder-type collars, and herbal collars that contain no pesticides (557). The skin-absorption collar is the one most likely to cause trouble for the dog. It operates on the principle that fleas all have to take a blood meal from the dog to live, and that they can be poisoned through the dog's bloodstream. The pesticide is taken in through the dog's skin and permeates the animal's system with enough poison to be fatal to the insects. Tests have been performed to determine whether this is also a health risk to the dog, but the results have been inconclusive so far, and the long-term effects of this method are still unknown. One real drawback for the absorption collars is that you have to be careful not to let the animal get wet—otherwise the amount of pesticide assimilated will increase and it may cause an irritation around the collar, not to mention a potential overdose of the insecticide. Collars that rely on flea powder are somewhat less effective because the flea must come in direct contact with the poison. The powder is circulated by the activity of the dog, and it's more effective in smaller dogs.

**553. Is it true that flea collars work because fleas have to migrate to the dog's face to drink from the dog's eyes and mouth?** No. Fleas live entirely on blood, and that's available just about anywhere on the dog's body.

**554. How good are the flea-killing disks that attach to the dog's collar?** These aren't bad. They use a vapor to control fleas, and they're safer than flea collars. However, they don't eliminate pests as thoroughly. They're better on smaller dogs because they use the same dispersion method that the powder flea collars do (552).

**555. *Are flea powders and sprays effective for controlling parasites?*** They're not as strong and thorough as flea collars, but they have a good residual action—one application lasts about a week. Like dips and collars, they're pesticides, so don't overuse them or apply them too often. If you have small children, it's wise to avoid powders and sprays.

**556. *Are there any flea-control methods that don't involve poisons?*** Yes. There are herbal collars and eucalyptus sprays as well as flea combs. Dietary methods can also be used. Large amounts of vitamin B generate an odor in the skin of dogs, people, and other mammals—it's undetectable to us, but repellent to biting insects. To give your dog a vitamin B boost, sprinkle a little brewer's yeast on his food. The daily dose for the summer season should be about one teaspoon per ten pounds of the dog's weight. Garlic is also said to help guard against fleas, although this hasn't been proven scientifically. Try chopping up a clove and adding it to the dog's meal —it can't hurt. Flea combs are available in most pet stores. They're useful as long as the dog's coat is thin enough to allow the fine teeth of the comb to pass through.

**557. *How good are natural herbal collars in preventing flea problems?*** They aren't perfect, but they do help. They can be combined with other organic methods to protect the dog without the use of pesticides. Herbal collars use a eucalyptus scent as a base, and their effectiveness lasts for about six weeks, which is short for a flea collar. Get some eucalyptus oil and mix it with water, then spray it on the dog in a light mist, rubbing it in with your fingers. If his vanity isn't too bruised by this strong, very uncanine aroma, it should help keep the fleas away. For a home-made flea collar without pesticides, mix up the same eucalyptus oil with a little cedar oil, citronella, and pennyroyal and soak it onto a length of twine; then seal it with some kind of silicone spray (hair spray will do).

**558. *Is there a new pill you can give dogs to protect them from fleas?*** Yes, and it's said to be the most effective method of flea control available. The pill is given each day, and it circulates the pesticide internally. This product may well be completely safe, but my advice is to wait and give it time to develop a safety record.

**559. *Isn't it dangerous to be giving a dog a pesticide in pill form?*** There's no evidence of toxicity so far in the tests that have been run on the product. However, it's only recently been developed, and it hasn't been proven safe in widespread public use. I only recommend it for animals in the southeastern U.S., where fleas have developed a resistance to most conventional controls.

**560. *My dog has a bump on his back. Could this be a tick embedded in his flesh?*** No. Ticks are always visible on the surface. What you *may* see is a swollen spot about the size of a pea that remains *after* a tick has bitten the dog and has been removed. This is harmless, and it should go away in about two weeks. If the bump becomes inflamed, take the dog to your vet because the area might become abscessed.

**561. *Do flea collars kill ticks?*** The ones that use pesticides do. Ticks usually embed themselves in the skin around the neck and head, where the flea collar's action is strongest. Unfortunately, natural herbal collars aren't a repellent for ticks; the best nonpoisonous way of controlling ticks is simply to remove them by hand. The best chemical control of both fleas *and* ticks is a dip every 10 days (550).

**562. What's the safest way to remove a tick?** Grab the tick between your thumb and index finger, or with a pair of tweezers, as close to the head as you can, and pull straight out, using a strong, constant force. You might leave the mouth parts of the tick in the dog's flesh, but this usually isn't a problem. It may cause a small inflammation that can be taken care of with three or four days of mild antiseptic cleansing. *Never* use gasoline or a burning match to remove a tick. This won't make the tick let go of the dog, and it may cause burns or other skin irritations.

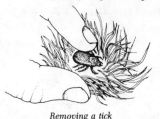

*Removing a tick*

**563. Isn't there a danger that ticks carrying Rocky Mountain Spotted Fever can infect a dog?** Yes. There's a danger to both dog *and* man from ticks carrying this disease. We can't catch the fever from a dog, but both dog and man can catch it from a carrier tick, and in rare instances the disease can be fatal. It occurs throughout the United States, and the symptoms in dogs are fever and a general lethargy. Some people believe that if they don't remove the head of a tick, their dog stands a greater chance of getting spotted fever, but this isn't true.

**564. Is it true that a tick bite can paralyze a dog?** A mild form of paralysis can result when a tick happens to bite over the rear end of a dog's spine. Enzymes secreted by the tick can cause nerve interference in the spinal cord, but the condition usually clears up when the tick is removed. This kind of paralysis can also affect people, but it's extremely rare.

**565. Are dogs bothered by lice?** Indeed they are. Lice are very contagious, and can be passed back and forth between dogs and humans—although lice are more common among people than among dogs. From a distance, lice may look like dandruff, but the flakes will be recognizable on a closer inspection. A dog with lice will itch and develop little red sores from the bites. Any good flea and tick shampoo can eliminate lice too.

**566. How can I tell if my dog has ear mites?** Dogs often catch ear mites from cats. An infestation of mites looks very much like an ear infection, and usually they can't be detected without examining a swab from the dog's ear under a microscope. The dog will shake his head from side to side and whine and scratch his ears again and again. In addition, the dog's ear wax will take on a dark color and begin to build up. Mites can be eliminated with medication from your vet.

**567. What could cause a round bald spot on my dog's head?** If the circle of bare flesh is getting wider, and the outer edges of it seem more irritated than the center, this could be the fungal disease called ringworm. The name is a misnomer; there's actually no worm attacking the dog. The condition is treated with oral and topical medicines. If you suspect that your dog has ringworm you should consult with your vet. Two other possible causes of such a condition are forms of mange, sarcoptic scabies and demodex (570).

**568. Can ringworm fungus spread to a person?** Yes. It's transmitted by direct contact and spreads rapidly. If you see signs of it, go to a dermatologist at once.

**569. *How can I tell if my dog has mange?*** Sarcoptic scabies, also known as red mange, is the itchy variety of this common skin condition. It's the work of a parasitic mite that's easily spread from dog to dog; it also attacks people. Because the condition is so communicable, the dog should be isolated until he's well again. Sarcoptic mites mostly attack the animal's elbows and neck, the skin around the eyes, and the tips of the ears. An infestation is probably the itchiest plague a dog can endure. A skin scrape by your vet can sometimes verify the presence of sarcoptic scabies, and treatment is lengthy but reliable. Some flea dips also kill scabies mites; check the package to find out if yours does, but consult your vet before using it because some pesticides are more toxic than others.

**570. *What are the signs of demodex?*** If your dog is young and has a bald spot on his fur he might have demodex, the nonitchy form of mange which is also caused by mites. Demodex can infest whole litters of puppies—and grows from a little, localized patch to a broad, serious problem. However, if your dog just has a little spot, it isn't a cause for alarm. Watch the affected area, and if it starts to widen, take the dog to your vet for tests. A small infestation can be ignored, but if the demodex begins to spread too far, drastic and sometimes dangerous treatment may be necessary. Sometimes even this fails, and when this happens, secondary infections and kidney failure usually kill the dog before too long. Demodex usually shows up when a dog is about three months old, and most of the minor spots of the infestation will clear up about the time the dog reaches puberty and develops an immunity to the mite. About ten percent of the serious cases also clear up at this point.

## Internal Parasites

**571. *I think my dog has worms. Should I get one of those over-the-counter worm products that you use once a month?*** Almost all of these products contain the same ingredient and are made to treat one kind of internal parasite, the roundworm. However, most adult dogs don't have roundworms; they're the plague of puppies (31). Some of the commercial wormers can also be dangerous if they're given to puppies. They're poisons for killing parasites, and too much of one of these products can cause vomiting, diarrhea, and even death. It's smarter to take stool samples to your vet and find out *exactly* what kind of worms your dog has.

**572. *How often should I have my dog checked for worms?*** Once a year, unless the dog has a history of worm problems. In that case I'd check for them twice a year.

**573. *Don't worms in a dog's digestive tract make him have to eat more than usual?*** This is only true for the tapeworm. All other worms cause an inflammation of the digestive system which reduces the dog's appetite. He just doesn't feel like eating.

**574. *My dog has been scratching his rear end along the ground and eating a lot more than usual. Is this a sign of worms?*** These are symptoms of a tapeworm infestation. The only other possibility is an impacted anal scent gland; this makes the dog scrub his rear end along the ground, but it doesn't affect his appetite (535). Most worms make a dog want to eat less, but tapeworms increase the animal's appetite because they eat part of the dog's food. If the dog has tapeworms you should be able to find them in his stool, and sometimes you can see them attached around the dog's anus. They look like little grains of rice, and they move with an accordianlike motion. You may have to look for them for a couple of days—they aren't always present in a bowel movement.

**575. *Is it hard to get rid of tapeworms?*** Yes. The tapeworm is certainly the hardest worm to kill. Only the most powerful wormers are of any use, and sometimes it's even necessary to give the dog enemas to kill the resilient head of the worm. This kind of worming requires a vet's care.

**576. *How does a dog pick up tapeworms?*** There are two kinds of tapeworms, one that comes from eating infected raw meat (usually a wild rodent), and a second that comes from fleas. The flea is the most common source of tapeworms in dogs. The infestation is produced this way: a flea larva will eat tapeworm segments, or eggs, and then hatch into an adult flea; then it lights on a dog and is picked off and eaten by the dog; inside the dog, the tapeworm egg hatches and matures, reproduces, and gives off new eggs which are then picked up by more flea larvae, completing the cycle. The rodentborne tapeworm is mainly a problem in rural areas, where it also poses a threat to human beings.

**577. *How big will a tapeworm get when it's inside a dog?*** Tapeworms grow up to two feet long in dogs; they can get as long as eight feet in a human.

**578. *How dangerous are roundworms?*** They can do some real damage to your dog. The roundworm follows a complex migratory route through the dog's body, from the stomach through the circulatory system and into the lungs. Once the worms are in the lungs, the puppy usually coughs them up and swallows them back down to the stomach and intestines. Damage to the lungs can cause inflammation and lead to pneumonia. Roundworms also weaken the animal and make him more susceptible to a variety of viruses and bacteria.(31)

**579. *Why do you have to treat a dog three times in a row with roundworm medicine?*** The worm follows a development cycle in the dog's body from larvae to adult. The medicine only kills adult roundworms, so you have to come back again two more times to get the larval worms as they develop. Waiting ten days between doses gives the larvae a chance to grow, but it kills them before they can reproduce and perpetuate the cycle.

**580. *Do older dogs get roundworms?*** Occasionally. They can pick them up from sniffing the feces of an infected animal—they get eggs on their nose and then swallow them by licking. The reason most older dogs don't get roundworms is that they develop an immunity with age. Roundworms are often transmitted to puppies because a pregnant dog may have a latent infestation that's been held in check by her immunity—but it becomes active as a result of her pregnancy.

**581. *What are heartworms?*** The heartworm is a round-shaped parasite that grows to a length of about eight inches. It lives, floating freely, in the right side of the dog's heart. A dog becomes infected with heartworms after being bitten by a mosquito that's carrying the parasite in its larval form.

**582.** *How does the mosquito pick up a heartworm larva in the first place?*   The mosquito becomes a heartworm carrier by biting and taking a blood meal from an infected dog. The dog's blood contains a microorganism called a microfilaria that becomes a larva. This is passed on to a second dog, where it becomes an adult, migrates to the dog's heart, and matures in about six months.

**583.** *How can you tell if a dog has heartworms?*   The only conclusive way is through a blood test. The worms reproduce microfilaria in the dog's bloodstream, and these can be seen in a blood sample. The external symptoms are a nonproductive cough and lethargy; the dog will easily become tired when she's exercising.

**584.** *Is it true that people can get heartworms?*   Heartworms are a serious problem for dogs, but it's extremely rare for them to infect people. Actually, people are probably bitten all the time by mosquitoes that carry heartworms, but we ordinarily have an immunity to this parasite. Parasites require a particular host in order to mature, and fortunately we aren't a host for heartworms. The cases that *have* occurred probably involved people with immunity problems.

**585.** *Do puppies have to be checked for heartworms?*   Pups less than six months old don't need to be tested because it takes that long for signs of the worm to show up.

**586.** *What's involved in the treatment of heartworms?*   The dog is hospitalized and an arsenical compound is injected in the animal's veins. This kills the worms and causes them to break up. The worms are in the right heart chamber and they stay there when they die so they can block the pulmonary vessels, causing a blood clot that blocks the blood from circulating to the dog's lungs. This is especially a danger if the worms have gone undetected for a long time. Another risk in the treatment is that the dog's body has to cleanse itself of the arsenical compound. This is done by the liver and kidneys, and the detoxification depends on whether these organs are working properly. If the dog has any liver or kidney problems, the compound could stay in the bloodstream a lot longer than intended and poison the dog. If the worms are found within a year, the problem is treatable and in most cases it will be successful, although there's *always* a risk of heart and lung damage. Any dog that undergoes this treatment will need a lot of rest for at least two months afterward.

**587.** *Couldn't heartworms be removed surgically?*   Surgery is only a last resort, and even then the dog requires drug treatment for the larvae in his system.

**588.** *Which kind of heartworm medicine is the best to use?*   The heartworm preventive drug comes in a variety of forms—liquid, tablets, and chewable—but they're all the same chemical, diethylcarbamazine citrate. It doesn't make a lot of difference what you buy, as long as it gets into the dog. However, I do suggest that you avoid putting the liquid in the dog's food; most dogs won't like the taste.

**589.** *How reliable is the preventive medicine for heartworms?*   There's very little likelihood that your dog will be infected with heartworms if he's receiving regular preventive medicine. However, the medicine isn't perfect, and there are some important reasons for having the animal tested at least once a year. First, the earlier the worms are detected, the more easily they can be eliminated. Second, if a dog has heartworms when he begins the preventive program, it could kill him when the larvae start to die because the burden of cleansing the system of the dead heartworm larvae can create a kind of toxic reaction that's more than the dog can take. Always check the dog for heartworms *before* beginning preventive treatment.

*590. Do you have to give a dog heartworm medicine year-round?*  In states that have a cold winter season that kills the mosquitoes, it's only necessary to give the dog medicine from April to December. In warmer climates, dogs need heartworm medication every day all year round because the mosquito population is never completely dormant. The potential for a heartworm infestation is much less in arid states, but it *has* been spreading. Originally, heartworms were only a major threat in the eastern U.S., particularly in the South, but the problem has spread west in recent years. Ask your vet or local kennel club about your area.

*591. What are the symptoms of hookworms?*  Hookworms are very small bloodsucking worms that grow to about a quarter of an inch in size and attach themselves to the walls of the dog's small intestine. They cause anemia, which can be very dangerous for puppies. Hookworms can be found in a fecal sample, but they usually can't be seen by the naked eye. The external symptoms to look for are a black, tarry stool and lethargy.

*592. What kind of treatment is available for hookworms?*  Over-the-counter wormers aren't available for this parasite because it's so difficult to get rid of. A hookworm infestation requires a vet's care.

*593. Can people get hookworms from dogs?*  People have their own kind of hookworm that's different from the one that infests dogs. By stepping in dog manure when you're barefooted, it's possible for you to pick up a dog hookworm larva, but the infant worm doesn't mature the way it does in a dog and will only migrate through the skin.

*594. How do you spot a whipworm infestation in a dog?*  There will be mucus in the stool that's generated by an inflamed colon. There will also be a loss of appetite and diarrhea, and in the morning the dog will vomit yellow bile. You can't see these parasites in the dog's stool. If you suspect that your dog may have whipworms, go to the vet to confirm their presence. Whipworms are the most persistent of the parasites (595). For this reason, the worming should be done by a vet.

*595. My dog is being treated for worms. Could these parasites have infested the ground in the yard where the dog stays?*  Yes, and this could be a problem, depending on the kind of worm the dog has and the type of yard you have. If the dog stays on concrete, all you have to do is hose it off regularly until after the dog is well. If you have a dirt yard, this *could* be a problem. When the dog is being treated for hookworms or roundworms you don't have much to worry about because the worms don't live long in the outside environment. Just clean up the dog's bowel movements daily until ten days after the last dose of wormer has been given. Whipworms are another matter. They can stay active in a yard for months, and they can even last through the winter if it's mild. To rid the yard of whipworms requires chemical treatment. Check with your vet about the commercial product available for this purpose.

# Miscellaneous Ailments

*596. What could make a dog start shivering with chill?* High-strung dogs often shiver when they're frightened. However, if the animal seems calm and the chills continue, this could be an indication that the dog has a fever. Take the dog's temperature (297), and if it's abnormal (288), take the dog to your vet.

*597. Do dogs suffer from anemia?* Yes. It usually occurs with other syndromes, and shows up through a blood test; the only outward sign may be pale gums. Anemia can be the result of blood loss, iron deficiency, or malignant lymphoma. Iron deficiency anemia can be cured with vitamin B-12 and iron supplements. Unfortunately, malignant lymphoma cannot be cured so easily. Efforts to treat this condition through chemotherapy have had little success (630).

*598. Is there a health danger if a male dog retains one or both testicles?* There are two forms of testicle retention, one harmless and one that can cause problems. Both are genetic defects, and they may affect one or both reproductive organs. An *inguinal testicle* remains alongside the penis. It's visible there, and it causes no particular health problem, although the temperature from the body tissues surrounding it will prevent it from producing sperm. If the testicle isn't visible in the scrotum or alongside the penis, it's most likely been retained in the abdomen. For reasons that we still don't clearly understand, testicles located in this area have a statistically higher risk of cancer. In this case, the safest thing to do is to have the dog neutered.

*599. What is the trouble if a dog's penis doesn't retract and seems to be causing the animal pain?* Sometimes the hair around the prepuce (the foreskin) folds in and irritates the inner tissues, causing an infection. When this happens, the dog's penis may be stuck out, and there could be a greenish discharge, groin pain, and red, inflamed skin. The dog will be continually licking the area, and he may be reluctant to urinate. This isn't a serious problem. Just wash the infected area with a mild antiseptic twice a day, and it should clear up in 5 or 6 days. You may also apply an antibiotic ointment. If the condition doesn't show signs of healing in 2 or 3 days, or if the dog is in a lot of discomfort, take him to your vet.

*600. What could make a dog's testicles swell up and become sore?* The dog's scrotum is covered with very sensitive skin. Contact with harsh soap, floor cleaners, or other irritants can all cause a condition known as scrotal dermatitis, in which the scrotum becomes enlarged, inflamed, and very painful. The dog may lick the area a lot, and this further aggravates the situation. It can even cause an infection to spread to the testicles. Other possible causes of testicular swelling are abscesses, tumors, and brucellosis (358), which causes chronic cycles of scrotal dermatitis.

# PART VI

# SERIOUS ILLNESSES

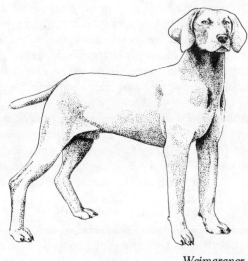

*Weimaraner*

## Hip Dysplasia
601-604

## Distemper
605-613

## Rabies
614-617

## Heart Disease
618-622

## Cancer
623-630

## Other Serious Illnesses
631-645

## Euthanasia
646-647

# Hip Dysplasia

**601. My dog has developed an odd, hopping kind of walk; it seems as if he can't bend his back legs. What could be the trouble?** This condition is called hip dysplasia. Dogs suffering from it have trouble standing up and lying down, and they walk with their back feet pointed outward and their knees together. Hip dysplasia is a genetic disorder. The hip joints become extremely arthritic, and the cartilage disappears as bone fills in until there's virtually no joint left at all. The condition usually shows up in a dog's x-rays when he's between 6 months and 2 years old, even though the dog may seem to walk normally. The physical signs of the disease can occur at any time. Hip dysplasia usually affects German shepherds and other large breeds such as retrievers, Irish setters, and huskies. It's not as common among the giant breeds. Among the large breeds, there's *one* that doesn't have this problem, and that's the greyhound, probably because of the dog's remarkable musculature.

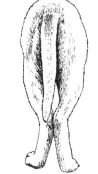

**602. How can I make sure my dog doesn't have hip dysplasia?** If you have a dog you're thinking of breeding, have an x-ray taken to make sure the animal doesn't have signs of hip dysplasia—this is the best way to reduce the prevalence of the disease. If you're buying a puppy, ask if the parents have been checked for signs of hip dysplasia. You may even be able to get certification of this by contacting the Orthopedic Foundation for Animals, 817 Virginia Ave., Columbia, Missouri, 65201. To obtain a certificate, a dog owner has to mail the foundation a set of x-rays of the dog's hips. The dog must be at least 2 years old at the time of the x-rays in order to be certified because signs of hip dysplasia don't always show up before then.

**603. What can be done for a dog with hip dysplasia? Is it curable?** There's no way to reverse the extent of the damage done by the disease, and no drug treatment that can do anything but treat the pain. However, there *are* two surgical techniques that can improve the dog's condition. Pectineomyotomy is a surgical method in which a ligament from the hip joint is severed. This is a controversial approach, and some veterinarians question whether it does any good at all. It's aimed at reducing the pain involved in movement, and the operation doesn't interfere with the joint. It *does* change the gait of the dog, loosening the structure of the joint and probably making the dog more comfortable in some cases. It seems to me that it's worth a try, especially since the other alternative is total replacement of the dog's hip, a procedure that's done only in severe cases. This operation is long, expensive, and complicated; it requires a specialist's knowledge and hospital facilities. The operation has been perfected over recent years, and it's reliable if it's done by an orthopedic specialist, but it's still so rarely performed that it's virtually unavailable in some parts of the country.

**604. What kind of home care can I give a dog that has hip dysplasia?** If a dog shows signs of dysplasia, don't run him too often and keep his walks short. Let the animal exercise himself; don't push him. You want the dog to be active, but not stressed. It's also a good idea not to let him sleep outside in cold, damp weather. When the dysplasia is particularly bad, give the dog aspirin for the pain (308), and if this doesn't work your vet can give the dog stronger medication.

## Distemper

**605. Does distemper cause a dog to become mean and start biting?** No. Distemper has nothing to do with a dog's temperament, and a distemper shot isn't given to prevent a dog from biting. Distemper is a viral disease that destroys the gut, brain, and lung tissue and wipes out the animal's ability to fight off other diseases. Dogs that have distemper usually die of pneumonia or some other bacterial infection. As a major dog disease distemper is diminishing because of the vaccinations that are available. Nonetheless, it's still the number one killer of young puppies.

**606. How is distemper spread?** Through contact with infected dogs. A dog picks up distemper by direct contact with the urine, feces, or mucus of an infected dog, or occasionally by airborne contact, although this is very unusual. An unvaccinated older dog may not have an active case of distemper, but he can still be a carrier of the virus. These dogs develop an immunity to distemper because they have encountered mild forms of the infection and survived it. However, without the vaccination, they can still get the serious form of the disease, although this rarely happens.

**607. If I get a new dog that hasn't been vaccinated for distemper, should I keep him away from other dogs?** Yes. Keep him isolated until he's safely vaccinated because other dogs may be carriers. If you get a dog that's older than eight weeks, he should have had at least one distemper vaccination. The only exception to this might be a dog you've gotten free from a private home. If you pay anything at all for a puppy, he should have had a minimum of one distemper vaccination.

**608. What are the symptoms of distemper?** In the pure sense of the word, there are almost no symptoms of distemper itself. The disease is a viral one that attacks and weakens the lungs, brain, intestines, and other organ systems. Most of the symptoms you see when a dog has distemper are the results of secondary bacterial invaders that move in on the weakened animal. Once this happens, you can look for a cough; vomiting; diarrhea; lack of appetite; and green, heavy mucus from the nose and eyes. In its final stages, there will be convulsions caused by brain damage. The seizures usually show up two weeks to a month after the first signs of distemper occur.

**609. What can I do at home for a dog that has distemper?** Be sure to clean the discharge of mucus from the dog's eyes and nose. This can cake up badly and make breathing difficult, and cleaning it also helps get rid of some of the infectious bacteria. Encourage the dog to eat, offering him mostly bland foods because his intestinal tract is infected—feed him cottage cheese, applesauce, boiled meat, chicken, and rice. It may even be necessary to force-feed the dog mashed food and liquids with an eyedropper. Also keep the dog in a comfortable place. He'll be undergoing enough stress without fighting cold weather or a lot of heat. MOST IMPORTANT: Be conscientious about giving the dog his antibiotics. Because of the highly contagious nature of the disease, the dog cannot be hospitalized. It will be up to you to provide the medication.

*610. Is there a cure for distemper?*   It *is* treatable with antibiotics and intravenous fluids. The recovery rate is about fifty percent. More important, it's almost completely preventable if the dog is given a series of inexpensive vaccinations. When a puppy is six to eight weeks old it should get a distemper shot, then another in two or three weeks, and a third in another two weeks. After that, just one shot a year until the dog is ten years old will protect him from this deadly virus.

*611. Our dog was diagnosed as having distemper and looked pretty bad for a while, but now he seems to be getting a lot better. Is the worst over?*   It may just have been a mild case, but distemper can also be very deceptive. The fever that accompanies the disease comes in two waves. This means that the dog will have a high temperature, which will drop back to normal for a while and then climb again. Sometimes this makes it look like the dog is getting better, and a couple of weeks may pass before the signs of neurological damage begin to show up. Don't stop the medication or let the dog go out of quarantine just because his condition seems to have improved. Wait, and consult your vet.

*612. Does distemper leave any permanent effects on dogs that recover from it?*   Yes. Often dogs that recover from distemper have suffered some degree of brain damage and nerve damage. This may show up as a kind of facial tic. If it's severe, the problem can usually be controlled with drugs.

*613. If a dog has a serious case of distemper, with brain damage, should he be put out of his misery?*   This depends on the dog's condition. Talk it over with your veterinarian. Some kinds of neurological problems can be controlled with drugs, while others could leave the animal badly handicapped and suffering.

## Rabies

*614. Is a vicious, biting dog more prone to rabies than a quiet one?*   No. Dogs of all temperaments are equally capable of contracting rabies. All that's necessary is for the dog to be bitten by a rabid animal. This can be another dog or a wild animal. Of course, if a dog has a tendency to roam, to fight with other dogs, and to chase wildlife, his chances of encountering a diseased animal are increased over that of a less active dog or one that's restricted by city li'

*615. Is there anything besides rabies that migh cause a dog to foam at the mouth?*   The dog could be simply panting very hard, o he may have eaten something with a very bitter taste. Of course, these will be *temporary* occurrences, and will not be accompanied by the other bizarre behavior associated with rabies.

*616. I was bitten by a dog, and I'm worried that he may have been rabid. How can I tell if he has this disease?*   First, try to find the owner to see if the dog has had his rabies shots (458). If the animal is actively infected with rabies and is capable of transmitting it (the disease can incubate in the dog's body for up to six months before it becomes communicable), the dog will come down with the signs of rabies within 10 days. Quarantine the dog and watch him carefully. There are two basic types of behavior associated with rabies—dumb and vicious. The dog may be affected with an extreme stupor, causing him to stand and stare for hours, or he may begin to wildly attack anything and everything, including inanimate objects. This is probably caused by hallucinations. Both kinds of rabies will be accompanied by an inability to swallow (which causes the dog's mouth to foam) and a kind of fear of water. This second symptom gave rise to the archaic name for the disease, "hydrophobia."

*617. Is there a cure for rabies?* No. A dog that's suspected of having rabies should be quarantined until the diagnosis is verified, but then the animal will have to be euthanized.

## Heart Disease

*618. Does heart disease affect some breeds more than others?* Yes, although it can affect any dog, heart disease is more prevalent among poodles, cocker spaniels, and beagles. It usually affects dogs over ten years old, and it's a product of genetics and old age, an inherited tendency that finally develops as the dog matures.

*619. Why does heart disease make a dog cough?* A dog with heart disease will have a dry, generally nonproductive cough at night or while she's exercising. This is related to the failure of the heart to pump blood efficiently, usually because a valve has stretched out of shape. When this happens, the heart tries to compensate by enlarging and sometimes pumping faster, and the rest of the body increases the volume of the blood by retaining salt. This is why people and dogs with heart disease must reduce their intake of salt. When the body retains salt, this creates an excess of fluid all over, including the lungs. This makes the dog cough, and it can eventually kill her by making it nearly impossible for her to breathe. The fluid is deep in the lungs, and it's extremely difficult for the dog to cough it up. This is why a persistent cough should not be ignored, particularly in an older dog.

*620. Besides coughing, what other symptoms of heart disease should I look for?* The dog may tire easily and have difficulty breathing. However, these are also symptoms of a heartworm infestation (583), so it would be wise to take the dog in for a checkup.

*621. Do dogs get heart murmurs?* Yes, they do. A heart murmur can have a number of different causes—it may be a genetic defect in the dog's heart, or it can be incidental and have no adverse effect on the animal's health. A heart murmur is also an early sign of heart disease, and it sometimes develops when a dog becomes anemic and the body strains to compensate for a lack of oxygen in the bloodstream. You can only hear a heart murmur with the aid of a stethoscope—it's a swishing noise between the beats of the heart.

*622. What kind of treatment is there for heart disease?* First, there are drugs: digitalis to strengthen the heart and diuretics to reduce the fluid in the chest. There is also a salt-free diet, using either special dog foods or home-cooked preparations. In addition, the dog's exercise can be limited under a veterinarian's supervision. With proper care, a dog with a bad heart can live out a normal lifespan.

# Cancer

**623. What kinds of cancer do dogs get?**   Skin tumors are the most common form of cancer in dogs. Dogs may also get mammary cancer; prostate cancer; leukemia; intestinal and stomach cancer; and liver, spleen, and bone cancer. The last occurs mostly in large breeds. Dogs very rarely get cancer that starts in the lungs, although sometimes cancer spreads to the lungs from other organs.

**624. What are the warning signs of cancer in a dog?**   In most cases, cancer in dogs is a slow deterioration that has very few external signs. The dog may not eat well, may lose weight, and have a poor-looking coat, but none of these are specific signs of cancer. They may well be caused by something much less significant. However, if one of these conditions goes on for a month or more, it would be wise to have the dog checked. The exceptions to this lack of visible warning signs are bone, mammary (628), skin (626), and lymph node cancers (531). Bone cancer usually affects a dog's legs, and this causes him to go lame. Less often, the cancer occurs in the ribs or skull bones, creating a firm, painful swelling on the bone. Bone problems such as these often appear in St. Bernards, Pyrenees, and Great Danes.

**625. What kinds of treatment are available for cancer in dogs?**   The same ones that are used to treat humans: cobalt treatments, chemotherapy, radiation therapy, and surgery. Unfortunately, the expense may be far too high to make some of them worthwhile. As with humans, the results vary according to the type of cancer, how early it's detected, and the age and condition of the dog.

**626. My dog has a lump on her skin. Could this be cancer?**   Dogs get a lot of skin tumors, and about eighty percent of them are benign, just cysts that are easily removed (188). If your dog has one or more skin tumors, have one removed and tested to find out if it's malignant. If it isn't, you can leave the rest of them alone, particularly if the dog is old and you don't want to risk problems with anesthesia, or if the tumors are small.

**627. Are there physical differences between benign and malignant skin tumors that I can look for?**   Yes. A malignant tumor will have abnormal skin above it, skin that's ulcerated and reddish or black. A malignant tumor also comes on rapidly, growing fast. Both benign and malignant tumors are usually found on the legs of big dogs, while they tend to develop around the anus of smaller dogs. A benign tumor around a dog's anus is called an adenoma. (188)

**628. What are the signs of mammary cancer?**   Mammary cancer is the leading type of cancer in female dogs, particularly in those that haven't been spayed or were spayed after they were a year old. It will appear as a large, firm lump, usually under or around one of the nipples. There's no pain until the lump gets very large. Female dogs also get benign tumors in their breasts, and the only sure way to know which type your dog has is for your veterinarian to remove the tumor and perform a biopsy. There's a general tendency of malignant tumors to grow more rapidly than benign ones, and this sometimes can indicate how serious a threat a particular growth might pose. If the lump stays small (the size of a pea) and doesn't grow rapidly (for instance, doubling in size in a month's time), then there's a good chance it is benign. But this is no sure guide. The lump should be removed and examined if the dog is young and healthy enough to undergo the surgery. If the lump is growing quickly, it should be removed, regardless of the animal's general health.

*629. What are the chances for survival if a dog has a malignant mammary tumor?* The chances are slim. The odds improve the sooner the lump is removed, but the cancer can spread to other parts of the body through the blood and lymph systems, and it usually attacks the lungs. If the cancer spreads to the dog's other breasts, it generally moves along the same mammary chain, the same side of the dog. The original tumor can also grow to such a size that in some cases surgery is a danger in itself. For all these reasons, it's important that *any* sign of trouble be checked as quickly as possible.

*630. Could my dog have leukemia?* Dogs occasionally get leukemia, but it isn't very common. There are a number of different forms of canine leukemia, and the name is a general term that's used whenever cancer cells are found in the animal's blood. In dogs, the cancer usually takes the form of lymphosarcoma, cancer of the lymph nodes (531); cancer of the spleen; or bone-marrow cancer (624). There is no cure, but the condition can be treated with chemotherapy, just as it is in humans, and in some cases the dog's life may be prolonged for quite a while.

## Other Serious Illnesses

*631. Don't poodles and collies have a congenital problem that can cause blindness?* Progressive retinal atrophy is the name of this syndrome, and it usually affects poodles. In many cases, it's first noticed in an early physical examination by a vet because signs of the problem can be seen in the eye with an ophthalmoscope before any traces of sight failure appear. It's an irreversible genetic problem that leads gradually to blindness. The condition may also be accompanied by cataracts. Collie eye anomaly is also genetic, noticeable through an eye examination at an early age, and irreversible. If you intend to buy a poodle or a collie, ask the owner if there's any history of these conditions in the dog's background.

*632. What are the signs that a dog is getting cataracts?* Cataracts result from a progressive loss of water from the lens of the eye, which causes it to become more and more crystalline, fibrous, and opaque. Cataracts are often confused with the hazy, gray sheen that develops in the lens of older dogs (186). This light discoloration isn't a cataract, just a normal symptom of aging. A *true* cataract begins as a white crys-

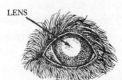
LENS

talline formation in the middle of a normally clear, black pupil. This is caused by failure of the lens to allow light to pass through; instead, it's being reflected back out of the eye. The crystalline spot will grow to full maturity, and in about six months it will block all light into the eye. You can tell the difference between a cataract and the aging haze on the surface of an old dog's eye by the fact that a cataract is very crystalline, not hazy, in appearance. Dogs can get cataracts at any age, and dogs can even be born with them. Cataracts have a number of causes, and sometimes they're interrelated with other diseases of the eye, and with diabetes (497). The only treatment is surgery; medicines don't help. If the dog can still see out of one eye, you may want to just let him adapt to the condition rather than go through the complex and costly operation that's necessary to restore a failing eye.

**633. What causes Addison's disease in dogs?**   This is the opposite of Cushing's disease (497). The dog's adrenal glands fail to produce enough steroids. The body loses salt, but there are no specific signs of illness until the latter stages of the disorder. Then the dog will become very weak, stop eating, and vomit repeatedly. Blood tests are required to confirm Addison's disease, and it's treated by the replacement of steroids with synthetic drugs.

**634. What is leptospirosis? Can people get it?**   Leptospirosis is a bacterial disease that attacks the kidneys. It's very contagious, and people *can* catch it. Humans usually come into contact with leptospirosis by swimming in ponds where unvaccinated dogs have been swimming. Fortunately, it's very rare for this to happen, and such contact is more common in the warmer, southern states. Leptospirosis is not ordinarily fatal, and it's treatable with antibiotics. Dogs pick it up from contact with infected urine. The symptoms are lethargy and some blood in the urine, although these symptoms may be so mild as to go unnoticed.

**635. Are kidney stones a problem with dogs?**   They can be, but only rarely. The signs are a pain around the lower back, difficulty urinating, and fever. Only a vet can accurately diagnose kidney stones, and they must be removed surgically. More commonly, dogs suffer from bladder stones or stones in the urethra (499).

**636. Is kidney failure curable?**   No. Unfortunately, there's no way to regenerate a failing kidney or arrest the impairment of a kidney. However, the dog's life can be prolonged by adjusting his diet.

**637. What kind of diet is needed when a dog is suffering from diseased kidneys?**   Your dog's diet should be devised under the supervision of your veterinarian, but basically the idea is to reduce the amount of protein. This is necessary because excess protein generates more nitrogen waste that must be excreted by the kidneys in the form of urea. If the kidney isn't functioning properly, this waste will keep building up and circulating in the body. Feed the dog low amounts of high-quality protein, such as eggs, along with carbohydrates in the form of rice or spaghetti. You should also add a vitamin and mineral supplement; this will help keep the toxins from building up. Even a healthy older dog shouldn't be fed as much protein as he received in his younger years (180).

**638. Don't dogs get a dangerous lung disease that's caused by a fungus? Can't they pass it on to people?**   There are four such fungal infections: blastomycosis, coccidioidomycosis (San Joaquin Valley Fever), cryptococcosis, and histoplasmosis. The San Joaquin strain is from California, and the rest occur chiefly in the Midwest. These are all very rare diseases for dogs, and they're even less likely to infect a person, although this is a possibility. These four diseases are severe, wasting illnesses marked by a chronic, downhill course. Each infects the lungs, but with no symptoms that would distinguish them from a case of pneumonia. They're spread through the inhalation of fungal spores that can be picked up anywhere in the infected dog's environment. These fungal diseases are curable, but the process is lengthy and a deep-seated case often proves fatal. There aren't many drugs that can fight an internal fungus, and none available today is a hundred percent effective. An infected animal also poses a public health risk. In most cases it's necessary to euthanize the sick animal to prevent a possible spread of the disease.

**639. How common is pneumonia in dogs, and what are its signs?**   It is unusual to see a dog with pneumonia because this disease is almost always a secondary infection that follows some other health problem. Most of the time, the disease that precedes it will call attention to the dog's ill health and the animal will receive medical care before pneumonia develops. The disease is generally associated with lingering bronchitis or the distemper virus. Pneumonia is a lung infection, either bacterial or viral. Its signs are fever; lethargy; a deep, usually nonproductive cough; and labored, shallow breathing. It's usually diagnosed by an x-ray and treated with antibiotics and vaporizing medication.

**640. Do dogs get jaundice?**   The thing to remember about jaundice is that it's a *symptom*, not a disease. Jaundice is the yellow tint seen in the skin as a result of liver problems. In dogs, the typical jaundiced color can be seen most easily in the gums and the exposed skin around the belly. The yellow color is caused by a build-up of impurities in the dog's bloodstream as a result of some interference with the liver—an infection, a blocked gall-bladder system, liver cancer, or congestion of the liver from heart disease or heartworms. In humans, jaundice is a symptom of hepatitis, but this isn't the case with dogs. If your dog has a jaundiced look, your veterinarian should examine him to discover the cause of the condition.

**641. I didn't know dogs got hepatitis. How serious a problem is it?**   Cases of hepatitis are rare in dogs today because of the vaccination that's now available (281). However, it remains a more prevalent syndrome in Bedlington terriers, apparently due to a genetic aberration. Other dogs are well protected with a yearly shot. Even if a dog *does* contract hepatitis, the disease isn't usually fatal. In most instances, it's a self-limiting illness that the dog will eventually throw off. The disease affects the liver, causing the dog to become lethargic; he'll lose his appetite and suffer from diarrhea. These outward symptoms are similar to a number of other disorders, and if your dog displays these signs you should have him examined by your vet.

**642. Is there such a thing as an epileptic dog?**   Yes, this does happen, and the cause isn't completely understood. There are two kinds of convulsive attacks, just as there are with humans—petit mal seizures and grand mal seizures. In neither type is the dog in any danger of choking on her tongue, which is a problem for people during grand mal seizures. *Petit mal* seizures are brief, and usually affect only a part of the dog's body. There may be a twitching spasm of a leg or some other muscle system for 30 to 60 seconds. Usually, the rear legs are affected. After the convulsion passes, the dog may be weak for a couple of minutes, and then she'll be back to normal. No treatment is necessary for petit mal seizures unless they begin to last longer and come more frequently. A dog may have an epileptic attack as often as every day or more, every week, or very rarely.

*Grand mal* seizures completely incapacitate the dog and send the entire body into convulsions. Usually the attack will be preceded by a small signal that a seizure is beginning. The dog may twitch or stare off blankly or snap at the air. After this, the dog will collapse—front and back legs paddling, throwing her head from side to side, salivating, sometimes vomiting, and losing bowel control. The seizure usually lasts from two to five minutes. When this happens, leave the dog alone. Place the animal on something soft, if necessary, and keep her away from ledges, stairs, and places where she could suffer a fall or bump her head. There's very little danger of the dog injuring someone who's trying to move her, although a person may be inadvertently bitten if he's accidentally caught in a jaw spasm. It's best just to isolate the dog in a safe place and leave her alone until the convulsions pass. When this happens, the dog will snap back to consciousness quickly, after a brief period of confusion.

A third and radical condition is an outgrowth of the grand mal seizure known as *status epilepticus*. In such a case, the dog does not stop convulsing. If a seizure goes on for 10 or 20 minutes, the dog should be taken *immediately* to your veterinarian for sedation. Anticonvulsant drugs aren't a cure for epilepsy, but they *are* a control, and usually a reliable one. However, canine epilepsy tends to grow worse over time and a dog with severe epilepsy may require so much of the drug that she's sedated 24 hours a day. In the case of an older dog with advanced epilepsy, it may be best to consider euthanasia.

**643. What else might cause convulsions besides epilepsy?** Brain damage from distemper, organophosphate pesticide poisoning, tetanus, brain tumors, head injuries, and even liver damage can all cause convulsions. In most cases, however, the difference is obvious. A dog that's suffering from any of these causes will not usually get up three minutes later and appear perfectly normal and then have the same problem six weeks or a year later. *That* is epilepsy.

**644. Do dogs have strokes like people do?** Dogs exhibit what appears to be a stroke syndrome, although the actual cause of this isn't understood. Unlike the strokes suffered by humans, canine strokes aren't caused by a blood clot in the brain. There's an initial convulsion, and the animal may pass out. After this, there's a temporary symptom of partial paralysis of one or more limbs. The stroke syndrome usually occurs in poodles and other small breeds, and will often resolve itself with proper medical management—rest, aspirin, and steroids, as well as some physical therapy that involves pulling and pushing the affected limb to keep the muscles in tone.

**645. Are dogs ever born with hemophilia?** Yes. Dogs are occasionally born with certain clotting deficiencies in their blood. This is a genetic factor, and it's more prevalent in purebred dogs. The signs usually appear when the animal is very young. The dog will bruise easily and bleed excessively if he's cut or scratched. If you see such signs, have your vet examine the dog.

## Euthanasia

**646. When a dog is gravely ill, at what point is it best to have him put out of his misery?** The decision to end a dog's life is a difficult one, no matter what the circumstances may be. Over the years, a dog can become an integral part of the family, and a person may grieve at his death as they would at the loss of any friend. Mourning the death of a pet is a natural and healthy reaction to a deeply felt loss. However, the situation is complicated by the fact that the owner is often called upon to decide *when* the dog should die. No one else can make this decision, and it means that the person must face some harsh realities during an emotionally upsetting time. For the sake of the owner's peace of mind, several things should be considered. Of course, the central question is the prognosis for the dog's future. It's easy to choose to have a dog put out of his suffering if he's unlikely to live through the night. Your vet should be questioned carefully about the animal's condition and the pain he may be subjected to by a disease or an injury.

A key concern should be the *quality* of the dog's life. When a dog's condition is irreversibly bad, but death isn't imminent (in the case of leukemia, or advanced spinal disease, for example), you should ask what the dog's future could be. It's important to remember that the natural lifespan of a dog is much shorter than our own. Consider the dog's age, and how long his life may be prolonged, even if the present critical problem wasn't an issue. Your own situation is just as important in making this kind of decision. If the dog needs nursing care and frequent medication, will you be able to provide it, or will there be long periods when no one is at home? How much can you afford to spend to postpone the dog's death, and what will be gained by you and by the dog in doing this? When you're faced with a painful, prolonged, expensive effort to fight off an incurable illness or injury, you shouldn't be burdened with guilt and doubt for not having chosen to postpone the inevitable. On the other hand, if the trouble, expense, and sacrifice aren't too great; if the bond between the owner and the dog is still strong (if there's still some communication there); and if the dog still seems to be strong in spite of his condition, then there may be something positive to be gained by waiting. (192)

*647. When a dog has died, what's the proper way to dispose of the body?* If you live in the country, you may want to bury the dog nearby. This is often against the law in cities, and in this case the SPCA will often pick up a dead animal or accept it for disposal if you bring it in. They sometimes also operate their own pet cemetery and crematory, or you could check the telephone directory for a private cemetery. Some cities also offer a removal and disposal service.

# APPENDIX

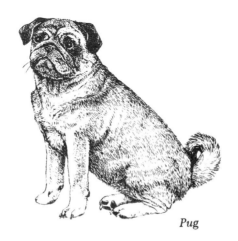

*Pug*

Annotated Bibliography
page 136

A First Aid Kit for Your Dog
page 138

Your Dog's Medical Record
page 140

# Annotated Bibliography

## Suggested Readings

Benjamin, Carol. *Dog Training for Kids.* New York: Howell Book House, 1976. $5.95, 150 pp.
An invaluable book that will help you insure a closer bond between your child and his or her pet. Most children can easily follow Ms. Benjamin's simple direction. A wonderful book.

Fiorone, Fiorenzo. *Enycyclopedia of Dogs.* New York: T. Y. Crowell, 1970. $25.00, 447 pp.
A beautiful book for anyone who loves dogs. Includes descriptions of specific breed characteristics and excellent photographs of every kind of dog.

Gerstenfeld, Sheldon. *Taking Care of Your Dog.* Reading, Massachusetts: Addison-Wesley, 1978. $6.95, 250 pp.
A good sourcebook on basic medical care for your dog, including reference charts to help you decide what ailments can be treated at home, and what ones need professional attention.

Hirshorn, Bernard. *Active Years for Your Aging Dog.* New York: Hawthorn, 1978. $12.50, 258 pp.
A valuable book that will help you make your pet's final years as rewarding as they can be.

Kohl, Sam, and Goldstein, Catherine. *The All-Breed Dog Grooming Guide.* New York: Arco, 1973. $9.95, 244 pp.
Kohl and Goldstein include charts and basic instructions detailing the grooming and care needed by most breeds. A good reference book for the amateur groomer.

Leob, Paul. *Complete Book of Dog Training.* New York: Pocket Books, 1974. $1.95, 253 pp.
An excellent book for anyone with a puppy or a problem pet. Leob gives sound advice on all aspects of dog training.

Lorenz, Konrad. *Man Meets Dog.* New York: Penguin, 1965. $2.95, 198 pp.
A world-renowned ethnologist provides interesting insights into the relationship between man and dog. A good mix of humor with a straightforward analysis of animal behavior.

Lydecker, Beatrice. *What The Animals Tell Me.* New York: Signet, 1977. $1.95, 147 pp.
A different approach to animal communication. Ms. Lydecker has a unique gift for expressing and understanding animal sensitivities. A good book for all animal lovers.

McGinnis, Terri. *The Well Dog Book*. New York: Random House, 1974. $10.00, 280 pp.
A well-organized, very complete book that concentrates on medical care.

Margolis, Matthew, and Siegal, Mordecai. *Good Dog, Bad Dog*. New York: Signet, 1973. $2.25, 250 pp.
This book covers the specific behavior problems found in 66 different breeds. The authors concentrate on techniques for obedience without punishment, and patience is the key.

Margolis, Matthew, and Swan, Catherine. *The Dog in Your Life*. New York: Random House, 1977. $12.95, 335 pp.
Margolis and Swan cover all aspects of canine care. A well-organized book that's a good reference tool.

Tortora, Daniel. *Help! This Animal is Driving Me Crazy*. Chicago: Playboy Press, 1977. $4.95, 306 pp.
An interesting case-by-case study of specific behavior problems, as well as good, sound advice to dog owners on how to cope with the problem dog.

In addition to the books listed above, here are three pamphlets that you may find helpful:

"How to Travel With Your Pet." Available free from the Humane Society, Dept. FB, 2100 L Street NW, Washington, D.C. 20037

"Puppy Rearing," by Peter Vollmer. An excellent booklet that can save you many aggravations in training your puppy. Available for $1 from Hills, P.O. Box 146, Topeka, Kansas 66601

"Touring with Towser." A listing of hotels and motels that accept animals. Available for $1 from Gaines, "TWT," Box 1007, Kankakee, Illinois 60901

# A First Aid Kit for Your Dog

Most of the medicine that's given to dogs is exactly the same as what's given to humans, so for minor problems, you shouldn't have to buy very many supplies that a well-equipped medicine cabinet wouldn't already have. Remember, though, that if your dog's condition hasn't improved within a day or so, you should substitute a veterinarian's care for these home remedies.

*Antacids (for vomiting).* Liquid preparations such as Pepto-bismol,® Maalox,® or Mylanta® will usually do the trick for a mild stomach upset. Give a child's dose to a small dog, and an adult dose to a dog that weighs up to 40 pounds (495). You can repeat the dose as often as every two hours.

*Aspirin.* Buffered products such as Ascriptin® or Bufferin® are best for dogs. Use one tablet per 20 pounds of the dog's weight, up to a maximum of two tablets (308). This dose can be repeated up to three times daily. Aspirin is useful for minor arthritis, fever, and irritating insect bites. CAUTION: Don't use aspirin on your dog for more than three days without consulting your vet.

*Antidiarrheal agent.* Nonprescription human medications such as Kaopectate® are usually effective in treating simple diarrhea in dogs. Use one tablespoon per 40 pounds of the dog's weight. You can repeat the dose every four hours (498). Breeds that are prone to bloat, such as Great Danes, will need to have plenty of human antigas tablets such as Di-Gel® on hand. You can give the dog two to three tablets after each meal. CAUTION: If diarrhea contains blood or has a foul odor, contact your vet.

*Antiseptic solution.* Over-the-counter drugstore antiseptics such as ST-37® and Camphophenique® do well for minor cuts and scrapes. ST-37® can also be used to treat ulcers in the mouth (296).

*Antiseptic powder and cream.* For a cut that's bandaged, an antiseptic such as Bacitiacid® works well in either gel or powder form. These will have longer and more concentrated action than other forms of antiseptics (296).

*Bandaging materials.* Cotton, sterile gauze, and "B-Z" adhesive tape should all be kept on hand for first aid use to stop bleeding quickly or to keep a wound clean (465).

*Cold capsules.* These usually provide temporary relief in cases of minor nasal and sinus congestion. Dogs over 30 pounds get an adult dose; those weighing 10 to 30 pounds get a child's dose; do *not* give cold capsules to dogs weighing under 10 pounds. Do *not* give cold capsules for more than two days without seeking veterinary advice.

*Cough medicines.* Follow the same directions for the dose as you would with cold capsules. Use only occasionally for minor coughs. If a cough persists for more than

72 hours, seek veterinary advice. CAUTION: Do *not* give your dog cough medicines that contain sedatives (codeine and phenobarbitol are the most commonly used ones).

*Constipation remedy.* If you're sure it's constipation, unflavored liquids such as Milk of Magnesia® will do, using a dose of one teaspoon per ten pounds of body weight. NOTE: Constipation is not the only problem that can cause your dog to strain (500). It's always best to check with your vet first.

*Eyedropper.* It's best to use one that's calibrated for exact measurements. *Never* use a glass eyedropper.

*Eyewash.* Boric acid eyewash will temporarily clean and sooth an irritated eye. You can use this up to three times daily. Do *not* use for more than two days. If the condition persists, call your vet (482).

*Glyoxide.* To prevent the build-up of harmful bacteria on the dog's teeth. If your dog has very bad teeth, use this once or twice a week with a cotton swab.

*Hemostats.* These surgical clamps may be hard to find, but they're extremely useful. They make plucking ears, pulling ticks, and removing objects from paws much easier.

*Ipecac.* Use as an emergency preparation to induce vomiting. Usually one teaspoon will do the job.

*Mineral Oil.* Good for cleaning a dog's ears.

*Motion sickness pills.* Human preparations such as Dramamine® usually work well. An hour before you start, give one tablet to dogs over 40 pounds and a child's dose to smaller dogs (169).

*Muzzle.* If your dog doesn't take well to being doctored, this can be an invaluable asset. Put on the muzzle before bandaging, clipping nails, plucking ears, and so forth. It will make the job easier for everyone concerned (145).

*Peroxide.* You can use ordinary three-percent hydrogen peroxide straight from the bottle to flush out wounds, open cysts, or clean ears (296).

*Petroleum jelly.* For removing tar, treating burns and scrapes, and lubrication.

*Rubbing alcohol (isopropyl alcohol).* Useful in cleaning ears or to keep a dog from chewing his paws. Apply lightly with a cotton ball.

*Styptic pencil or powder.* This will help stop a bleeding nail in a hurry.

*Thermometer.* Make sure you have a pediatric rectal thermometer. When you need to take the dog's temperature, be sure you lubricate the thermometer well with petroleum jelly (297).

# YOUR DOG'S MEDICAL RECORD

NAME_____

BIRTH DATE_____

BREED_____SEX_____

IDENTIFYING MARKINGS & COLOR_____

_____

SOURCE & DATE ACQUIRED_____

_____

*Photo*

VETERINARIAN_____

ADDRESS_____

EMERGENCY PHONE NUMBER(S)_____

## MEDICAL & SURGICAL HISTORY

VACCINATION HISTORY       DATE

   *Distemper*

   *Hepatitis*    }   __   __   __   __   __   __   __

   *Parainfluenza* }

   *Rabies*     __   __   __   __   __   __   __

WORMING_____

HEARTWORM CHECK_____

OVARIOHYSTERECTOMY or CASTRATION (Date)_____

## VETERINARY CARE & NOTES

_____

_____

_____

_____

_____

*This form may be photocopied for repeated use.*

# INDEX

NOTE: *Numbers in Index refer to
entries rather than pages.*

# A

abortion, 356
  brucellosis and, 358
  shot for, 320
abnormality, congenital, 394–395
abrasion, 469
abscess, of anus, 535
  of lymph node, 531
  swollen testicle and, 600
  tick bite and, 560
  of tooth, 515–516
accident, automobile, 443, 450, 454–455
  emergency treatment for, 443–494
  shock and, 451
achondroplasia, 394
Addison's disease, 633
adenoma, 627
adrenal gland, disease of, 633
afterbirth, eating of, 385, 388
age, new puppies and, 15
  old. *See* old dog.
  physical signs of, 256
age equivalency, dog and human, 243
aggressiveness, 245
  biting and, 236
  castration and, 333
aging. *See also* old dog.
  cataract and, 632
  dental care and, 189
  heart disease and, 618
  lifespan and, 243
  skin problems and, 187-188
  special care and, 180–192
airplane travel, 172–174
alcoholic beverages, 85
  as antidote, 488
allergy, of dog, 527–529
  coughing and, 525
  feeding bowl and, 148
  foot and, 532
  signs of, 527
  treatment for, 528
  to dog, 23
American Kennel Club, 18, 355
amniotic sac, 379
ampicillin, use of, 486
amputation, 546

anal scent gland, 251
  abscess of, 534–535
  impaction of, 574
anconeal process, ununited, 541
anemia, 597
  eye condition and, 283
  flea bites and, 547
  heart murmur and, 621
  pulse and, 291
anestrus, heat cycle and, 340
angle-pronged collar, 142
animal fat, care of coat and, 109
animal shelter, 5, 9
  adoption from, 19
ankle, arthritis and, 190
antacid, 308
antibiotic powder, 533
antibiotics, distemper and, 609–610
  ear infection and, 135
  food and, 305
  gum disease and, 141
  human, 307
  topical, 296
  use of, 486
antidote(s), poisoning and, 488
  universal, 490
antifreeze, poisoning by, 488
antiseptic, bite wounds and, 459
  kinds of, 296
anus, abscess of, 534
  atresia, 394
  tapeworm and, 574
  tumor and, 627
appetite, excessive, 87
  false pregnancy and, 361
  loss of, 312
  pain and, 282
  tapeworm and, 574
  whelping and, 372
  worms and, 573
arsenic, poisoning by, 488
arthritis, exercise and, 162
  hip dysplasia and, 601
  kneecap and, 540
  old dog and, 190
  rheumatoid, 545
artificial respiration, 446
  drowning and, 481

# Index

artificial respiration *(cont'd)*
  electric shock and, 480
ash content, dog food and, 79
aspirin, arthritis and, 190
  back pain and, 543
  dosages of, 308
asthma, 522
  coughing and, 520
atresia anus, 394
attack dog, 238
automobile, chasing after, 217
automobile accident, 443
  assessment of, 450
  examination after, 454–455
  moving dog from, 443
automobile travel, 169–171

# B

baby (human), puppy and, 197
  dog and, 199–200
baby aspirin, use of, 308
baby teeth, 256–257, 512
back, fracture of, 473
  pain in, 542–544
  sores on, 530
back ailment, obesity and, 93
backpacking trip, 177
bacteria, breath and, 141
  old dog and, 189
bald spot, causes of, 567
bandage, compound fracture and, 472
  on foot pad, 478
  pressure, 465
barking, as communication, 252
  confinement and, 54
  training against, 223, 224
  puppy and, 57
basset hound, back pain and, 542
  eyelid of, 504
bathing, 115–118
  dry, 117
  flea control and, 549–551
  procedure for, 116
beagle, back pain and, 542
  children and, 193
  heart disease and, 618
  puppy and, 149
Bedlington terrier, hepatitis and, 641
beer, as antidote, 488
bee sting, treatment for, 491
begging, discipline and, 63
behavior, aggressive, 236
  bone-burying, 248

behavior *(cont'd)*
  cage and, 51, 54
  castration and, 332–333
  chasing animals, 216
  chasing cars, 212, 217
  communicative, 252
  destructive, 207
   puppy and, 62
  digging and, 218
  of Doberman pinscher, 237
  ear infection and, 134
  eating and, 98, 239
  epileptic, 642
  false pregnancy and, 361
  heat cycle and, 341
  high-strung, 231
  hostile, 238
  housebreaking and, 230
  human contact and, 20
  incontinent, 231
  maternal, 419–423
  nesting, 249
  old dog and, 183
  possessiveness, 240
  postpartum, 389
  problematic, 207–240
   professional training and, 67
  puppy and, 13, 15. *See also* puppy.
  rabies and, 616
  second dog and, 25
  sense of sight and, 264
  sexual, 349, 352–353
   mounting and, 228
  spaying and, 327–328
  submissive, 233
  territoriality and, 229
  unfriendly, children and, 196
  urination and, 287
  whelping and, 372
bicycle, chasing, 212
  leash and, 167
birth. *See* whelping.
birth control, 319, 321, 334. *See also* spaying
  *and* castration.
  castration and, 330
birth defect, 394–395
birth process, children and, 204
bite, from insect, 491
biting, 238
  distemper and, 605
  force of, 177
  human and, 458
  muzzle and, 145, 209
  puppy and, 65
  rabies and, 616
  treatment for, 459

*Numbers in Index refer to entries rather than pages.*

142

bladder, infection of, 499
 ruptured, 454
bladder control, training for, 231
bladder stones, 499
 ash content of food and, 79
blastomycosis, 638
bleach, poisoning by, 488
bleeding, control of, 465–466
 cut foot and, 465
 heat cycle and, 341
 internal, signs of, 291, 447
 nail clipping and, 124–125
 tourniquet and, 466
 treatment for, 444
 vaginal, mating and, 347
blindness, genetic, 631
blink response, 445
bloat, 88, 89
blood, disease of, 645
 human compatibility and, 279
 in stool, 286
blood clot, heartworm and, 586
blood pressure, gum color and, 447
 stress and, 292
 taking of, 299
blood types, 278
boarding, 179
boat, travel by, 176
body odor, cause of, 530
bone, burying of, 248
bone(s), broken, 473
  splint and, 474
 diseases of, 537–544
bone cancer, 624, 630
bones, eating and, 83
boots, 153
boredom, 207
bowel movement, difficulty in, 500
bowl, puppies and, 436–437
 types of, 148
brain damage, convulsions and, 643
 distemper and, 608, 612–613
 heat stroke and, 461–462
 temperature and, 289
breast, cancer of, 628–629
 infection of, 405
  whelping and, 401, 404
breath, foul-smelling, 141, 511, 515–516
 old dog and, 189
 shortness of, accident and, 455
breathing. *See* respiration.
breech position, 375
breed(s), 1, 3, 8. *See also specific kind.*
 aging and, 180
 allergy to, 23
 back pain and, 542–543

breed *(cont'd)*
 biggest, 276
 boat travel and, 176
 Caesarean section and, 377
 children and, 193
 city and, 1
 collapsible trachea and, 521
 exercise and, 159
 fastest, 272
 "fear biting" and, 236
 heart disease and, 618
 hemophilia and, 645
 hip dysplasia and, 601
 intelligence and, 241
 knee problem and, 540
 lifespan and, 243
 mating and, 355, 359
 sight failure and, 631
 smallest, 274
 stroke and, 644
 tallest, 273
 watchdog and, 27
breeder, buying from, 5
breeding, heat cycle and, 342
 hip dysplasia and, 602
 preparation for, 346
 small dogs and, 275
 studs and, 343
 veneral disease and, 358
bronchitis, pneumonia and, 639
brucellosis, 358
 mating and, 346
 scrotal dermatitis and, 600
brushes, types of, 101
brushing, 100. *See also* grooming.
 method of, 102
 puppy and, 48
bulk food, old dog and, 180
bulldog, achondroplasia and, 394
 Caesarean section and, 377
 eyelid of, 504
bull mastiff, size of, 276
bull terrier, aggressiveness of, 245
burn, chemical, 479
 electric, 480
 minor, 478
 treatment of, 477
butter, coat and, 109

# C

Caesarean section, 376–377
cage, 151

*Numbers in Index refer to entries rather than pages.*

cage *(cont'd)*
  car travel and, 171
  outdoor, 168
  puppy and, 50–54
"caged dog syndrome," 232
cage-type muzzle, 145
cairn terrier, 1
calcium, eclampsia and, 408
  pregnancy and, 363–364
  puppy and, 33
  whelping and, 401
calmness, training for, 231
calories, puppy and, 33
campgrounds, 178
cancer, 623–630
  inguinal testicle and, 598
  mammary, 628–629
    spaying and, 326
  old age and, 188
  skin, 626–627
    nose and, 526
  spaying and, 323
  swollen lymph node and, 531
canned food, 69
  puppy and, 33, 35
carnasal tooth, 515
carrying case, 151
castration, 331–333
  housebreaking and, 229
  inguinal testicle and, 598
  mounting and, 228
  puppy and, 29
  roaming and, 214
  spaying and, 330
cat, as companion, 26, 210
  intelligence of, 242
cataract, 506, 632
  old dog and, 186
  retinal atrophy and, 631
cavity, dental, 139
cemetery, 647
cervical disk disease, 537
chain choker, 142
chain leash, 146
chasing, discipline and, 217
  territoriality and, 212
check-up(s), veterinary, 280
  old dog and, 181
  postpartum, 384, 401
  puppy and, 30
chemical, caustic, burn from, 479
chemical poisoning, 488
chemotherapy, cancer and, 625, 630
cherry eye, 502
chewing, of furniture, 62
  toys and, 154, 156

chewing gum, removal of from coat, 111
chew toys, destructiveness and, 62
Chihuahua, 1
children, 193–206
  behavior of, 203
  breeds and, 193
  dipping and, 551
  new dog and, 21, 22
  sex of dog and, 10
  stray dog and, 202
chills, 596
chlorophyll, heat cycle and, 357
choker, leash training and, 226
choker collar, 142
choking, toys and, 155
  treatment for, 463
  use of collar and, 144
cholesterol, 92
chow, aggressiveness of, 245
city, breed and, 1
claws, back, 123
  caring for, 119–127
    bleeding and, 124–125
    medical problems and, 120
    puppy and, 48
cleft palate, 394
clippers, mat removal with, 110
  types of, 122
clipping, of nails, 119–127
  poodles and, 100
clock ticking, puppy and, 53
coat, aging and, 18
  diet and, 105
  general care of, 100–118
  general health and, 284
  healthy appearance of, 105
  postpartum shedding of, 409
  of puppy, 12
    diet and, 33
  shedding of, 103–104
  vitamins and, 81
coccidioidomycosis, 638
coccidiosis, kennel and, 43
cocker spaniel, children and, 193
  city and, 1
  heart disease and, 618
cold, common, 517
cold capsules, 308
colitis, diarrhea and, 496
collapsible trachea, collar and, 142
  coughing and, 521
  harness and, 144
  leash training and, 226
collar, electric, 225
  Elizabethan, 313, 469, 533
  flea, 552–553

*Numbers in Index refer to entries rather than pages.*

collar, flea *(cont'd)*
  herbal, 556–557
  ticks and, 561
  types of, 552, 554
puppy and, 40
spiked, 143
training, 226
types of 142–143
collie eye anomaly, 631
"collie nose syndrome," 526
colorblindness, 265
colon, inflamed, 496
coma, death and, 445
comb, flea, 556
  wide-toothed, 101
commercial dog food, alternatives to, 71
common cold, 517
communication, barking and, 252
competition, males and, 24
  territory and, 29
compound fracture, 472
confinement, housebreaking and, 61
  of puppy, 51
  roaming and, 214
  urination and, 250
conjunctivitis, 503–504
consciousness, coma and, 445
constipation, 500
  treatment for, 308
convulsion, distemper and, 608
  epileptic, 642
  nonepileptic, 643
  poisoning and, 488
  stroke and, 644
copulatory lock, 349
coughing, 520–525
  heart disease and, 619
cough medicine, liquid, 308
cream rinse, bathing and, 116
crematory, 647
crossbreed, 8
cruciate ligament, 475
cryptococcosis, 638
Cushing's disease, 633
  urination and, 497
cut. *See* wound *and* injury.
cyst, benign, 626
  old age and, 188

## D

dachshund, 275
  back pain and, 543
dalmatian, 193

dandruff, 106
  puppy and, 12
deafness, 510
  human, dogs and, 255
death, 646–647
  signs of, 445
debarking, 225
decay, dental, 139
defecation, difficulty in, 500
  laxative and, 308
dehydration, appearance of eye and, 283
  signs of, 293
  vomiting and, 495
delivery. *See* labor.
demodex, 570
  balding and, 567
dental care, 139–141. *See also* teeth.
  old dog and, 189
dental disease, check-up for, 280
dermatitis, scrotal, 600
destructiveness, 62
  training and, 207
dew claws, 120, 126–127
  removal of, 401
DHLP vaccination, 280
diabetes, cataract and, 632
  signs of, 497
diaphragm, hernia of, 454
diarrhea, chronic, 496
  mild, 498
  treatment for, 308
Dieffenbachia, poisoning by, 489
diet, bladder stones and, 499
  carnivorous, 73
  dandruff and, 106
  dental care and, 140
  diarrhea and, 498
  distemper and, 609
  exercise and, 96
  flea control and, 556
  heart disease and, 622
  kidney disease and, 637
  old dog and, 180
  postpartum, 399
  pregnancy and, 363
  protein and, 70
  shedding and, 104
  skin condition and, 108
  starvation, 94
  vegetarian, 77
  of weaned puppies, 442
diethylcarbamazine citrate, heartworm and, 588
dieting, 95
  commercial dog food and, 97
diet pills (human), 310

*Numbers in Index refer to entries rather than pages.*

digestion, 75
  of rawhide, 156
  weaning and, 435
  worms and, 573
digestive system, obstruction in, 464
digging, discipline for, 218
digitalis, 622
dipping, flea control and, 549–551
  sarcoptic mites and, 569
  ticks and, 561
discharge, uterine, 403
discipline. *See also* training.
  collar and, 142
  destructiveness and, 207
  hitting puppy and, 56
  housebreaking and, 61
  indoor urination and, 229
disease. *See also specific kind.*
  Addison's, 633
  of adrenal gland, 633
  of cervical disks, 537
  congenital. See *defect, genetic.*
  dental, 141
  distemper and, 605
  of eye, 631–632
  fungal, 567
    of lung, 638
  of hip, 538, 601–604
  immunity of newborn from, 400
  kennel and, 43
  of kidney, 634
  of lung, 639
  in mouth, 511
  pet shop and, 6
  periodontal, 511
  regional, 175
  respiratory, 517–525
  roundworm and, 578
  veneral, 358
disk, vertebral, disease of, 537, 542
distemper, 605–613
  convulsions and, 643
  coughing and, 520
  kennel and, 43
  pneumonia and, 639
  puppy and, 12, 414
  symptoms of, 608
  treatment for, 610
  vaccination for, 281
    kennel and, 179
distress, respiratory, 446
diuretics, 622
Doberman pinscher, behavior of, 237
  temperament of, 247
  as watchdog, 27
docking, of tail, 430

dogfight, dangers of, 246
  first aid and, 459
  new dog and, 29
  responding to, 456
dog food, bulk quantities of, 72
  commercial, alternatives to, 71
  dieting and, 97
  puppy and, 440
  types of, 69
doghouse, 150
dominance, 25, 29
  nipping and, 65
dosage, of antibiotics, 486
  of aspirin, 308
drain cleaner, poisoning by, 488
drooling, 261, 516
  Doberman pinscher and, 237
drowning, resuscitation from, 481
dry bath, 117
dry food, 69
  puppy and, 33, 35
dryness, of coat, puppy and, 12
dumbcane, poisoning by, 489

## E

ear(s), caring for, 131–137
  cleaning, 132
  cropping, 137–138
  floppy, 258, 259
  infection of, 134
  object in, 493
  problems with, 507–510
  puppy and, 12, 426
  shape of, hearing and, 258
  swelling of, 507
eardrum, 133
ear mites, 134, 566
eating. *See also* feeding *and* diet.
  illness and, 312
  speed of, 239
eclampsia, signs of, 408
  whelping and, 401
edema, pulmonary, 480
eggs, puppy and, 36
egg white, 80
elbow, crippled, 541
  injury of, 536
electric collar, 225
electric shock, 480
  heart massage and, 448
Elizabethan collar, 313, 469, 533
emergency, first aid for, 443–494

*Numbers in Index refer to entries rather than pages.*

emergency *(cont'd)*
    automobile accident, 443, 450, 454
    bleeding, internal, 447
    bone, broken, 471–475
    breathing and, 446, 455
    burn, 477–479
    choking, 463–464
    dog bite, to human, 458
    dogfight and, 456, 459
    drowning and, 481
    drugs and, 487
    ear problem, 493
    electric shock and, 480
    eye problem and, 482–483
    fishhook and, 485
    foot, cut in, 465
    frostbite, 494
    heartbeat and, 448–449
    heat stroke, 460–462
    insect bite and, 491
    poisoning, 488–490
    shock, 451
    smoke inhalation, 476
    snakebite, 492
epilepsy, 642
estrogen, abortion and, 356
estrus, heat cycle and, 340
ethylene glycol, poisoning by, 488
eucalyptus, flea control and, 556, 557
euthanasia, 192, 646
    birth defects and, 394–395
    distemper and, 613
    epilepsy and, 642
    lung disease and, 638
    rabies and, 617
evisceration, 315
exercise, 158–168
    car travel and, 170
    diet and, 96
    feeding and, 90
    heart disease and, 622
    hip dysplasia and, 604
    kennel and, 179
    old dog and, 182
    pregnancy and, 365
expenses, new dog and, 2
eye(s), blink response of, 445
    cataract of, 632
    color of, 429
    distemper and, 608–609
    general health and, 283
    grooming and, 113
    medicine and, 306
    of newborn, 393
    object in, 482
    old dog and, 186

eye *(cont'd)*
    problems with, 501–506
    puppy and, 426–429
    redness of, 504–505
    retinal atrophy and, 631
    socket and, 483
    tearing and, 283
eye-contact, dog and human, 420
eyedropper, use of, 306
eyelid, 266
    conjunctivitis and, 504
    third, 502
eyesight, 264–265

## F

fallopian tubes, tying of, 324
false pregnancy, 361
fang, upper, 512
fat, care of coat and, 109
    general health and, 92
    puppy and, 33
fatty tumor, old dog and, 188
fear, of human, 232–233
    shivering and, 596
    training against, 221–222
"fear biting," 236
feces, color of, 286
    eating of, 208
        training and, 234–235
    roundworms and, 205
    taking sample of, 301
    tapeworm and, 574
feeding, 69–99. *See also* diet.
    cage and, 52
    exercise and, 90, 160
    old dog and, 180
    postpartum, 399
    puppy and, 33–38, 435–442
    weaning and, 432–435
feeding bowl, 148, 436–437
feet, 128–130. *See also* foot pad.
female, heat cycle of, 340
    male and, 10
    sexual maturity of, 335
femoral artery, pulse and, 298
femoral head necrosis, 538
femur, kneecap and, 540
fence, electrification of, 219
fertility, loss of, 336
    periods of, 340
fetus, death of, 384, 403
fever, distemper and, 611
    nose and, 285

*Numbers in Index refer to entries rather than pages.*

fever *(cont'd)*
  shivering and, 596
  ticks and, 563
fighting, 456
  breeds and, 245
fire, smoke inhalation and, 476
first aid, 443–494. *See* emergency.
  supplies for, 295
first-stage labor, 372
fishhook, removal of, 485
flatulence, diet and, 86
flea(s), 547–558
  bathing and, 548
  shorthaired dog and, 11
  tapeworm and, 576
flea-bite allergy, 527
flea collar, 552–553
  herbal, 556–557
  ticks and, 561
flea control pill, 558–559
flea powder, 555
flea soap, use of, 550
flea spray, 555
flies, ear bites from, 508
flu, 517
fluid, in chest, 619
foaming, of mouth, 615
food, medicine and, 305
foot pad, bandage on, 478
  burn of, 478
  cut in, 465
  exercise and, 164
  frostbite of, 494
  injury and, 128–130
  protection of, 153
  soreness of, 532
  sweat and, 261
formula, commercial, 411
    weaning and, 432–433
four-in-one vaccination, 281
fracture, auto accident and, 454
  in leg, 471–472
  signs of, 473
  splint and, 474
frostbite, treatment of, 494
"full heat," 340, 341
fungus, lung disease and, 638
  ringworm, 567–568
fur. *See* coat.

## G

gagging, 521
garlic, flea protection and, 84, 556

gas, in stomach, 88
gasoline, poisoning by, 488
gastric torsion complex, 88
genitalia, infection of, 358
German shepherd, city and, 1
  "fear biting" and, 236
  hip dysplasia and, 601
  as watchdog, 27
gestation, period of, 362
glands, reproductive, 270
glaucoma, cataract and, 506
  signs of, 505
golden retriever, children and, 193
  eyelid of, 504
  flaky coat and, 107
grand mal seizure, 642
grass, eating of, 253
Great Dane, cancer and, 624
  lifespan of, 244
  size of, 276
greyhound, hip dysplasia and, 601
  speed of, 272
groin, pain in, 599
groomer, professional, 100, 114
grooming, 100–118
  bathing and, 116
  dandruff and, 106
  ear infection and, 136
  eye and, 113
  of nails, 119–125
  pregnancy and, 367
  tools for, 101
growth, cancerous, 627
  old dog and, 187–188
growth plate, 17
guard dog, 27
gum(s), anemia and, 597
  disease of, 141
  infection of, 511, 516
  internal bleeding and, 447

## H

hair. *See also* coat *and* grooming.
  ear infection and, 136
hallucination, rabies and, 616
hand feeding, 312, 411, 421
handling, of injured dog, 452–453
  puppy and, 13–14, 47, 424–425
harness, 144
  leash training and, 226
hashish, ingestion of, 487
health, annual check-up for, 280
  condition of coat and, 284

*Numbers in Index refer to entries rather than pages.*

health *(cont'd)*
  flea collars and, 552
  general, 280–293
  new puppy and, 12
  postpartum, 402–408
hearing, ear infection and, 509
  sense of, 258
hearing-ear dog, 255
heart, worms and, 586
heart attack, 292
  human, dog and, 254
heartbeat, abnormal, 291, 449
  location of, 445
  rate of, 290
heart disease, 618–622
  coughing and, 520
  obesity and, 93
heart massage, 448
  electric shock and, 480
heart murmur, 621
heartworm(s), 581–590
  coughing and, 520
  exercise and, 162
  heart disease and, 620
  medication for, 588–590
    preventive, 418
    travel and, 175
  symptoms of, 583
heat, exercise and, 163
heat cycle, 335–342
  breeding and, 342
  chlorophyll and, 357
  false pregnancy and, 361
  frequency of, 339
  mating and, 348
  signs of, 341
  spaying and, 325, 328–329
  stages of, 340
  time of, 335
heat stroke, 460–462
  airplane travel and, 172
  doghouse and, 150
  obesity and, 93
  temperature and, 289
Heimlich maneuver, 463
hemophilia, 645
hepatitis, 641
  appearance of eye and, 283
  vaccination for, 281
herbal flea collar, 556–557
  ticks and, 561
hermaphroditism, 270
hernia, diaphragmatic, 454
  perineal, 500
  umbilical, 416
herpes virus, 414

hip, arthritis in, 190
  disease of, 538
  injury of, 536
hip dysplasia, 601–604
  certification and, 602
  exercise and, 162
  studs and, 343
  vitamin C and, 82
histoplasmosis, 638
hitting, discipline and, 56
hives, 529
hookworm(s), 591–593
  medication for, 592
hostility, 238
  maternal, 421
housebreaking, 59–61
household, cat and, 26
  new dog and, 25
  new puppy and, 28
  puppy and, 19, 49
  urinating in, 229
  watchdog and, 27
husky, aggressiveness of, 245
  exercise and, 159
  hip dysplasia and, 601
hydrocephalus, 395
hydrophobia, 616

# I

ice, protection of feet from, 128
identification, tattoo and, 41
immunity, vitamin C and, 81
  nursing and, 400
inbreeding, 345
incision, surgical, 315–317
incontinence, 185, 231
inertia, uterine, 375
infant, human, dog and, 198
infection, of bladder, 499
  of conjunctiva, 503
  of cyst, 188
  distemper and, 606
  in ear, 131, 134, 509
    ear mites and, 566
  of eye, puppy and, 427
  fungal, 638
  of gums, 511, 516
  in joint, 470
  of lung, 639
  of lymph node, 531
  mammary, 405
  of penis, 599
  postsurgical, 315

*Numbers in Index refer to entries rather than pages.*

infection *(cont'd)*
  respiratory, 518
    appearance of eye and, 283
    puppy and, 12
  of skin, 533–535
    puppy and, 44
  smoke inhalation and, 476
  of tear gland, 502
  temperature and, 289
  of tooth, 515–516
  uterine, 403
    whelping and, 401
  wound and, 313
inguinal testicle, 598
inhalation, of smoke, 476
injury. *See also* wound.
  auto accident and, 443, 450, 454–455
  carrying dog with, 452
  emergency treatment for, 443–494
  of eye, 482
  on foot pad, 465
  fracture and, 473
  human, from dog, 458
  of joint, 536–541
  in leg, 475
  of ligament, 471
  temperament and, 453
  of tendon, 471
inner ear, 133
insect. *See also specific kind.*
  bite of, 529
    treatment for, 491
  ear and, 508
insemination, artificial, 354
instinct, paternal, 397
intelligence, of breeds, 241
  dog v. cat, 242
intestine, distemper and, 608
  virus of, 495
I.Q., 241
Irish setter, children and, 193
  eyelid of, 504
  flaky coat and, 107
  hip dysplasia and, 601
Irish wolfhound, height of, 273
iron, anemia and, 597

**J**

jaundice, 640
jaw, fracture of, 473
  auto accident and, 454
jogging, 162–165

joint, disease of, 545
  hip, disease of, 601–601
  injury of, 536–541
  sprain of, 470
joint mice, 539
jumping up, training and, 64

**K**

kennel, 179
  disease and, 43
kennel club, buying from, 5
kennel cough, 523–524
  vaccination for, 281, 524
kerosene, poisoning by, 488
kidney disease, 634
  diet and, 637
  heartworm and, 586
  urination and, 497
kidney failure, 636
  burn and, 477
kidney stones, 635
knee, injury of, 475
  sprain of, 536
kneecap, disease of, 540

**L**

labor, complications in, 375, 381
  delay in, 375, 383–384
  onset of, 371
  signs of, 372
Labrador retriever, children and, 193
lameness, causes of, 470
  old dog and, 190
laxative, 308, 500
lead-based paint, poisoning by, 488
leash, bicycling and, 167
  jogging and, 165
  training and, 146, 226
    puppy and, 40
leather leash, 146
leg, amputation of, 546
  fracture in, 471–472, 474
  limp of, 540–541, 601
    cancer and, 624
  pain in, 471
lens, dysfunction of, 632
leptospirosis, 634
  vaccination for, 281
leukemia, 630

*Numbers in Index refer to entries rather than pages.*

Lhasa apso, brushing and, 100
　city and, 1
lice, 565
license, 42
　fee for, 2
licking, prevention of, 313
　soreness and, 532–533
lifespan, 243
　breeds and, 244
　cataract and, 632
　diet and, 180
　euthanasia and, 646
ligament, injury of, 471
　　knee and, 475
　strained, 470
light, shedding and, 103
limb, amputation of, 546
　fracture in, 471–472, 474
liquid medicine, administration of, 304
litter, orphaned, 410
　runt of, 412
　size of, 368, 384
liver, cholesterol and, 92
　disease of, 93
　　heartworm and, 586
　hepatitis and, 641
　jaundice and, 640
long-distance running, 162–165
longevity, 243, 244
longhaired dog, choice of pet and, 11
　grooming and, 100, 112
lost dog, 215
LSD, ingestion of, 487
lung, auto accident and, 454
　cancer of, 623
　collapse of, 455
　distemper and, 608
　fluid in, 480
　fungal disease of, 638
　infection of, 518, 639
　roundworm and, 578
　smoke inhalation and, 476
　water in, 481
luxating patella, 540
lymph node, cancer of, 630
　swollen, 531
lymphoma, anemia and, 597
lymphosarcoma, 531

# M

malamute, aggressiveness of, 245
male(s), competition and, 24

male *(cont'd)*
　female and, 10
　paternal instinct and, 397
　sexual maturity of, 335
　stud service and, 343–344
malocclusion, 513
　dental disease and, 141
malpresentation, 375
mammary cancer, 628
　spaying and, 323, 326
mange, 569
　balding and, 567
　nonitchy, 570
marijuana, ingestion of, 487
massage, of heart, 448
　electric shock and, 480
mastitis, 405
　treatment for, 406
　whelping and, 401
mating, 346–355
　abortion and, 356
　age for, 335
　duration of, 349–351
　preparation for, 346
mats, grooming and, 101, 110
mat splitter, 101
maturity, sexual, 335
meat, diet and, 73
　raw, 74
　weaning and, 435
medical care, home, 294–318
medical costs, new dog and, 2
medical records, 294
medication, administration of, 303–306
　　liquid, 304
　　oral, 303
　antibiotic, 486
　common, 308
　flea control and, 549–555
　food and, 305
　human, 307–310
　record of, 294
　shampoo and, 116
metestrus, heat cycle and, 340
microfilaria, heartworm and, 582–583
milk, mammary, 400
　　infection and, 406
　　insufficiency of, 407
　　spaying and, 329
　　weaning and, 432–433
　puppy and, 36
milk fever, whelping and, 401
mineral oil, 308
mite(s), ear, 134, 507, 566
　sarcoptic, 569
mixed breed, 8–9

*Numbers in Index refer to entries rather than pages.*

mood, pain and, 282
"morning after" shot, 356
mosquito, heartworm and, 581–582, 590
mother, surrogate, 421
motion sickness, 169
mounting, 228, 352
 castration and, 333
mouth, disease of, 511
 drooling and, 261, 516
 fishhook in, 485
 foaming of, 615
 hygiene of, 262
mouth-to-mouth resuscitation, drowning and,
 481
 electric shock and, 480
mucus, in stool, 286
murmur, of heart, 621
muscle, strained, 470
mutt, lifespan of, 244
 mating and, 359
 temperament and, 4
muzzle, barking and, 223
 discipline and, 208–209
 types of, 145
 vicious dog and, 457

# N

nail clipping, bleeding and, 124–125
 puppy and, 48
nails, caring for, 119–127
 medical problems and, 120
neck, fracture of, 473
 injury of, 537
nervousness, 231
 fear and, 233
nervous system, distemper and, 612
nesting, 249
neutering. *See* castration *or* spaying.
newborn, artificial respiration for, 392
 breathing of, 379
 eating of, by mother, 389
 emergence of, 373–374, 378–384
 hand-feeding and, 407
 handling of, 396
 orphaned, 410
 other dog and, 398
 physical problems of, 394–395
 security of, 369
new dog, shopping for, 1–27
Newfoundland, lifespan of, 244
newspaper training, puppy and, 60
new tricks, old dog and, 183
nictitating membrane, 266

nictitating membrane *(cont'd)*
 inflammation of, 502
nipple(s), grooming and, 367
 male dog and, 269
 milk production and, 407
 number of, 268
noise, fear of, 218, 220–222
nose, distemper and, 608–609
 general health and, 285
 irritation of, 518
 soreness of, 526
 sweat and, 261
nuclear sclerosis, 186
nursing, immunities and, 400
 problems with, 423
 spaying and, 329
nutrition. *See also* diet *and* feeding.
 pregnancy and, 363
 puppy and, 33–38
 types of dog food and, 69
 weaning and, 432–435
nylon choker, 142
 leash training and, 226
nylon leash, 146

# O

obedience, training and, 209
obedience instruction, professional, 67
obesity, 93, 95
 starvation diet and, 94
odor, mouth and, 141, 511, 515–516
oil, skin care and, 108
old age, breeds and, 243–244
old-age warts, 187–188
old dog, arthritis and, 190
 cataract and, 632
 check-up and, 181
 common afflictions of, 185–190
 coughing and, 520, 619
 diet and, 180
 exercise and, 182
 hearing and, 510
 heart disease and, 618
 lifespan and, 243
 new tricks and, 183
 puppy and, 191
 rheumatism and, 190
 roundworm and, 580
 suffering of, 192
organophosphate pesticide, poisoning by, 488
orphan, care of, 410
osteoarthritis, 190
outdoor run, 168

*Numbers in Index refer to entries rather than pages*

outdoors, puppy and, 55
ovariohysterectomy, 322. *See* spaying.
overbite, 513

# P

pain, 192, 282
  abdominal, poisoning and, 488
  in back, 542-544
  broken leg and, 472
  defecation and, 500
  examining dog with, 453
  in groin, 599
  hip dysplasia and, 604
  limping and, 470-471
  in neck, 537
  in scrotum, 600
paint, ingestion of, 488
  removal of from coat, 111
palate, cleft, 394
pancreatitis, 92
  eating feces and, 234
  obesity and, 93
panting, heat stroke and, 461, 462
paper training, puppy and, 60
parainfluenza, vaccination for, 281
paralysis, stroke and, 644
  ticks and, 564
parasite(s), children and, 205
  eating feces and, 234
  external, 547-570
  internal, 571-595
parvovirus, 413
patella, luxating, 540
pavement, exercise and, 158
  jogging and, 129, 164
paw. *See also* foot pad.
  size of, puppy and, 17
pectineomyotomy, 603
pedestrians, chasing, 212
Pekinese, achondroplasia and, 394
  eye of, 483
pelvis, fracture of, 473
    auto accident and, 450, 454
penis, 349
  infection of, 599
perineal hernia, 500
periodontal disease, 141, 511
  sneezing and, 518
permanent teeth, 46, 256-257, 512
personality. *See* temperament.
perspiration, 261
  heat stroke and, 461

pesticide, flea control and, 552, 555
  ingestion of, 488
  use of, 549-551
pet cemetery, 647
petit mal seizure, 642
pet shop, buying from, 6-7
philodendron, poisoning by, 489
phosphorus, puppy and, 33
pill, administration of, 303
  birth control, 319
  flea control and, 558-559
"pink eye," 503
placenta, eating of, 385, 388
  expulsion of, 384-385
  retention of, 403
plants, poisoning by, 489
plaque, bad breath and, 189
  stains from, 511
plastic, allergy to, 148
pneumonia, 638-639
  coughing and, 520
  distemper and, 605
  kennel cough and, 523
  roundworm and, 578
  smoke inhalation and, 476
poinsettia, poisoning by, 489
pointer, shorthaired, 193
poison(s), 488-490
  convulsions and, 643
  fleas and, 552
  plants and, 489
  snakebite wound and, 492
Pomeranian, 226
poodle, 1, 226
  blindness and, 631
  children and, 193
  collapsible trachea and, 521
  grooming and, 100
  heart disease and, 618
  hip disease and, 538
  human allergy and, 23
  intelligence of, 241
  tear duct of, 501
  toy, knee problem of, 540
    litter of, 368
population, control of, 328
porcupine, quill of, removal of, 484
possessiveness, training and, 240
postnasal drip, sneezing and, 519
postpartum care, 401-409
powder, flea control and, 552, 555
powder bath, 117
pregnancy, 360-368
  abortion and, 320, 356, 358
  age and, 338
  duration of, 362, 371-372

*Numbers in Index refer to entries rather than pages*

pregnancy *(cont'd)*
  false, 361
  loss of coat during, 409
  prevention of, 319, 324
  roundworm and, 580
  spaying and, 329
  worming medicine and, 366
presentation, of newborn, 375, 378
pressure bandage, 465
preventive medicine, 280–293
proestrus, heat cycle and, 340, 341
progressive retinal atrophy, 631
prolapsed rectum, of puppy, 417
prolapsed uterus, 390
prolapsed vagina, 391
prostate gland, infection of, 500
protein, 70
  kidney disease and, 637
  old dog and, 180
  pregnancy and, 363
  puppy and, 33
  vegetarian diet and, 77
pseudohermaphroditism, 270
pug, city and, 1
  eye of, 483
pulse rate, 290
  taking of, 298
punishment, discipline and, 56
puppy. *See also* newborn.
  acquisition of, 12–19
  cage and, 50–54
  collar and, 40
  demodex and, 570
  dehydration in, 495
  diet and, 33–38
  diseases of, 413–414
  distemper vaccination and, 607, 610
  early development of, 15
  ears of, 426
  eyes of, 393, 426–429
  feeding, 435–442
  flea bites and, 547
  grooming and, 48
  hand-feeding of, 411
  handling of, 396, 424–425
  heartworm and, 585
    preventive medicine for, 418
  hip dysplasia and, 602
  hookworm and, 591
  housebreaking and, 59–61
  human baby and, 197
  I.D., tattoo and, 41
  learning tricks and, 66
  maternal neglect of, 423
  new home for, 28, 29
  old dog and, 191

puppy *(cont'd)*
  personality and, 13
  prolapsed rectum of, 417
  roundworm and, 571, 578
  security of, 369
  signs of health of, 12
  skin infection and, 44
  sleep and, 45
  special care of, 28–55
  toys and, 39, 62
  training and, 29, 56–68, 425
  umbilicus of, 415–416
  use of bed and, 149
  veterinarian and, 30
  vitamin supplements and, 81
  weaning of, 432–442
  weather and, 16
  worms and, 31
puppy stressing, 425
purebreds, 1
  advantages of, 3
  mating and, 355, 359
  temperament and, 4
Pyrenee, cancer and, 624

# Q

quarantine, distemper and, 611
  rabies and, 616, 617
quill (porcupine), removal of, 484

# R

rabies, 614–617
  airline travel and, 174
  dog bite and, 458
  vaccination for, 177, 280
radiation, cancer and, 625
rash, allergy and, 525
rat poisoning, 488
rawhide toys, 156
recognition, sense of smell and, 251
rectum, prolapsed, 417
red mange, 569
reproduction. *See also* behavior, sexual.
  Caesarean section and, 376–377
  organs of, 270
respiration, artificial, 392, 446
  drowning and, 481
  electric shock and, 480
  difficulty in, 446

*Numbers in Index refer to entries rather than pages*

respiration *(cont'd)*
  diseases of, 517–525
  newborn and, 379
respiratory infection, puppy and, 12
responsibility, of children, 194–195
resuscitation, mouth-to-mouth, 392, 446
    drowning and, 481
    electric shock and, 480
retina, atrophy of, 631
retriever, exercise and, 159
  hip dysplasia and, 601
reverse sneezing, 519
rheumatism, 545
  old dog and, 190
rib, fracture of, 473
ringworm, 568
  balding and, 567
roaming, 213
  castration and, 333
  discipline and, 214
Rocky Mountain Spotted Fever, ticks and, 563
rope training, 211, 227
roundworm(s), 578–580
  children and, 205
  medication for, 571
  puppy and, 31, 571
  treatment for, 32
rubber ball, 154, 157
running, 162–165
  leash and, 227
runt, of litter, 412
rupture, of bladder, 454

# S

salivary gland, inflammation of, 516
salivation, 261
salmonellosis, diarrhea and, 496
salt, foot irritation and, 128
  heart disease and, 619
saluki, speed of, 272
San Joaquin Valley Fever, 638
sarcoptic scabies, 569
  balding and, 567
scent, association and, 52
  skunk and, 118
scent gland, anal, abscess of, 534-535
  impactation of, 574
schnauzer, hermaphroditism of, 270
  human allergy and, 23
scooting, 535
  tapeworm and, 574
scratching, ear infection and, 134

scrotum, swollen, 600
season, allergy and, 527
  bathing and, 115
  heartworm and, 590
  shedding and, 103
sebaceous cyst, 188
seborrhea, 106, 530
  ear care and, 131
second-stage labor, 373
sedatives, cold medicine and, 308
  human, 309
seizure, distemper and, 608
  epileptic, 642
  nonepileptic, 643
semi-moist patties, 69
senility, 185
  hearing and, 510
sex. *See also* behavior, sexual.
  choice of dog and, 10
  new dog and, 24
sex organs, 270
sexuality, spaying and, 328
shampoo, 116
  dandruff, 106
  flea, 551
shedding, 11, 103-104
sheepdog, brushing and, 100
shivering, 596
shock, electric, 480
    heart massage and, 448
  medical, treatment for, 451
shorthaired dog, choice of pet and, 11
  grooming and, 100
shoulder joint mice, 539
sick room, 311
sight, loss of, 631
  sense of, 264
silent whistle, 147
simple fracture, in leg, 472
sinus, infection of, 518
skin, allergy and, 527-528
  cancer of, 526
  demodex and, 570
  disease of, dandruff and, 106
    old age and, 187
  dry, diet and, 108
  flaking, 530
  infection of, 533
    puppy and, 44
  lump on, 534
    old age and, 188
  mange and, 569
  tumor, 623
    benign, 626
    malignant, 627
  vitamins and, 81

*Numbers in Index refer to entries rather than pages*

skin-absorption collar, 552
skunk scent, bathing and, 118
sleep, old dog and, 184
    puppy and, 45
    urination and, 250
sleeping, with children, 201
smell, recognition and, 251
    sense of, 258, 260, 264
smoke, inhalation of, 476
snacks, 99
snakebite, treatment for, 492
sneezing, 518
    reverse, 519
    sinus problem and, 527
sniffing, as greeting, 251, 252
snort, 519
social order, 13, 25, 29
socket, loose eye and, 483
sore. *See also* abscess, injury *and* wound.
    on back, 530
    treatment of, 533
spaying, 322-330
    abortion and, 356
    age and, 338
    birth control and, 319-320
    castration and, 330
    false pregnancy and, 361
    mammary cancer and, 628
    temperament and, 421
sperm, castration and, 333
spiked collar, 143
spleen, cancer of, 630
splint, use of, 474
sprain, in joint, 470
springer spaniel, children and, 193
    exercise and, 159
starvation diet, 94
status epilepticus, 642
St. Bernard, cancer and, 624
    children and, 193
    drooling and, 516
    eyelid of, 504
    lifespan of, 244
    litter of, 368
    size of, 276
sterility, 337
steroids, Addison's disease and, 633
    allergy and, 528
    water consumption and, 497
stitches, surgical, 314-318
    first aid and, 467
stomach, fever and, 285
    overeating and, 88
    upset, 495
stones, in bladder, 499
    in kidney, 635

stool, color of, 286
    sample of, 301
    tapeworm and, 574
storm, fear of, 221
strain, in leg, 470
strangers, human, fear of, 232
stray dog, approach to, 202
street noise, fear of, 222
stress, blood pressure and, 292
    diarrhea and, 496
stretcher, makeshift, 473
stroke syndrome, 644
strychnine, poisoning by, 488
stud service, 343-344
submissiveness, 25, 29, 233
sunburn, 526
suppository, 308
surgery, aftermath of, 315
    cancer and, 625
    orthopedic, 603
    suturing and, 314-315
swallowing, difficulty in, 616
    of foreign object, 464
sweater, 152
sweating, nose and, 285
swimmer syndrome, 394
swimming, 161
swollen joint, 470

# T

table begging, discipline and, 63
table scraps, 98
tail, docking of, 138, 401, 430
tangle splitter, 101
tapeworm, 574-577
    appetite and, 573
    fleas and, 547
    life cycle of, 576, 579
    treatment of, 575
tar, removal of from coat, 111
tartar, 140
    aging and, 256
    check-up for, 280
    periodontal disease and, 141
tattoo, identification of puppy and, 41
tears, draining of, 283
tear duct, 501
tear gland, infection of, 502
teeth, 512-513,
    abscess of, 515-516
    age of dog and, 256

*Numbers in Index refer to entries rather than pages*

teeth *(cont'd)*
 baby, 512
 bad breath and, 189
 care of, 139-141
 cleaning, old dog and, 189
 gum disease and, 141, 511
 loss of, 46
 number of, 257
 occlusion of, 513
 permanent, 512
 plaque stains on, 511
 tartar and, 140-141, 280
teething, 46
temperament, 4
 castration and, 332
 children and, 193
 distemper and, 605
 of Doberman pinscher, 247
 heat cycle and, 341
 male v. female, 10
 pain and, 282
 possessive, 240
 puppy and, 13
 rabies and, 614
 spaying and, 327
 studs and, 343
temperature, body, 288-289
 distemper and, 611
 heat stroke and, 460, 462
 normal, 288
 nose and, 285
 taking of, 297
 whelping and, 372
tendon, injury of, 470-471
terrier, 275
 children and, 193
 "fear biting" and, 236
 human allergy and, 23
territoriality, 212-213
 competition and, 29
 stress of, 292
 urination and, 229, 287
testicle, retention of, 598
 swollen, 600
tetanus, convulsions and, 643
tetracycline, use of, 486
thermometer, use of, 297
third eyelid, 266
 dehydration and, 283
 inflammation and, 502
thunder, fear of, 221
thyroid gland, coat condition and, 107
tick(s), 560-564
 dipping and, 549
 removal of, 562
 shorthaired dog and, 11

"the tie," 349
tongue, electric shock and, 480
tonsilitis, 514
tooth. *See also* teeth.
 abscess of, 515-516
toothpaste, 141
tourniquet, snakebite wound and, 492
 use of, 465-466
toy breeds, city and, 1
 "fear biting" and, 236
toys, 154-157
 behavior and, 62
 puppy and, 39
trachea, collapsible, collar and, 142
  coughing and, 521
  harness and, 144
  leash training and, 226
tracheobronchitis, 523
 coughing and, 520
 kennel and, 43
 puppy and, 414
 vaccination for, 524
training, cage and, 51, 151
 car chasing and, 217
 collar and, 142, 226
 incontinence and, 231
 leash and, 146, 226
 methods of, 66
 muzzle and, 145
 old dog and, 183
 problem dog and, 207-240
 professional, 67
 puppy and, 29, 56-68, 425
 silent whistle and, 147
 use of rope and, 211
 watchdog and, 27
training leash, 40
tranquilization, air travel and, 173
 car travel and, 171
 excitabilty and, 231
 fireworks and, 220
 grooming and, 114
transfusion, 278, 279
transmissible venereal tumor, 358
travel, by airplane, 172-174
 by boat, 176
 by car, 169-171
 regional disease and, 175
trench mouth, 511
tricks, teaching, 66, 183
tumor, fatty, 188
 mammary, 628
 skin, 623
  benign, 626
  malignant, 627
  old age and, 187

*Numbers in Index refer to entries rather than pages*

# U

umbilical cord, 385, 387-388
umbilical hernia, 416
umbilicus, of puppy, 415-416
underbite, 513
ununited anconeal process, 541
urination, auto accident and, 454
  difficulty in, 499
  excessive, 497
  excitement and, 231
  frequency of, 287
  incontinent, 185
  territoriality and, 229
urine sample, 300
uterine inertia, 375
uterus, infection of, 403
    whelping and, 401
  prolapsed, 390
  removal of, 322. *See* spaying.
  retention of fetus in, 384

# V

vacationing, 177-178
  travel and, 169-176
vaccination, annual, 280
  for distemper, 281, 607, 610
  for hepatitis, 281
  for kennel cough, 281, 524
  leptospirosis, 281
  parainfluenza, 281
  rabies, 177, 280
vagina, prolapsed, 391
  whelping and, 382
vasectomy, 334
vegetables, feeding of, 78
vegetarian diet, 77
venereal disease, 358
venom, poisonous, 492
vertebrae, disease of, 537, 542
viciousness, muzzle and, 457
  rabies and, 614, 616
virus, antibiotics and, 486
  corona, 413
  distemper and, 606
  herpes, 414
  intestinal, 495
  puppy and, 413
  respiratory, 518
  venereal, 358
vision, 264

vision *(cont'd)*
  cataract and, 632
  of color, 265
  loss of, 631
  of puppy, 428
vitamin(s), puppy and, 33
  supplements of, dandruff and, 106
    diet and, 81
    shedding and, 104
vitamin B, flea control and, 556
vitamin C, 82
  bladder infection and, 499
vitamin D, pregnancy and, 364
vocal folds, 271
  removal of, 225
vomiting, causes of, 495
  mild, 498
  poisoning and, 488
  treatment for, 308
vulva, heat cycle and, 341

# W

walking, dogfights and, 166
  exercise and, 158
  housebreaking and, 59, 230
  training and, 226
wart, old dog and, 187
watchdog, 27
  training puppy and, 58
water, consumption of, excessive, 497
  fear of, 616
  heat stroke and, 461-462
water on the brain, 395
"water sac," 372, 379
wax, in ear, 131
  check-up for, 280
  infection and, 134
weaning, 432-442
  period of, 441
weather, airplane travel and, 172
  arthritis and, 190
  exercise and, 163, 164
  longhaired coat and, 112
  paper training and, 60
  puppy and, 16
weight, 93
  feeding and, 91
  measurement of, 302
  reduction of, 95
weimaraner, exercise and, 159
whelping, 371-388

*Numbers in Index refer to entries rather than pages*

whelping *(cont'd)*
   age and, 338
   Caesarean section and, 376-377
   preparation for, 369
   spaying and, 326, 329
   supplies for, 370
whelping box, 369, 380, 431
whippet, speed of, 272
whipworm(s), 594
   backyard and, 595
   vomiting and, 495
whiskers, 263
whistle, silent, 147
worm(s), 205, 571-595. *See also specific kind.*
   check-up for, 572
   diarrhea and, 496
   environment of, 595
   flatulence and, 86
   puppy and, 31-32
worm medication, pregnancy and, 366
wound. *See also* emergency *and* injury.
   antibiotics and, 486
   bandage and, 465, 472, 478
   of eye, 482
   of foot, 465, 532
   human, from dog, 458
   licking of, 313
   minor, treatment of, 469
   snakebite, 492
   stitching of, 467-468
   treatment for, 444
wrist, arthritis and, 190

# Y

yeast, brewer's, flea protection and, 84
Yorkshire terrier, city and, 1
   size of, 274

*Numbers in Index refer to entries rather than pages*